PANDORA'S
Book of Sexual Fantasies

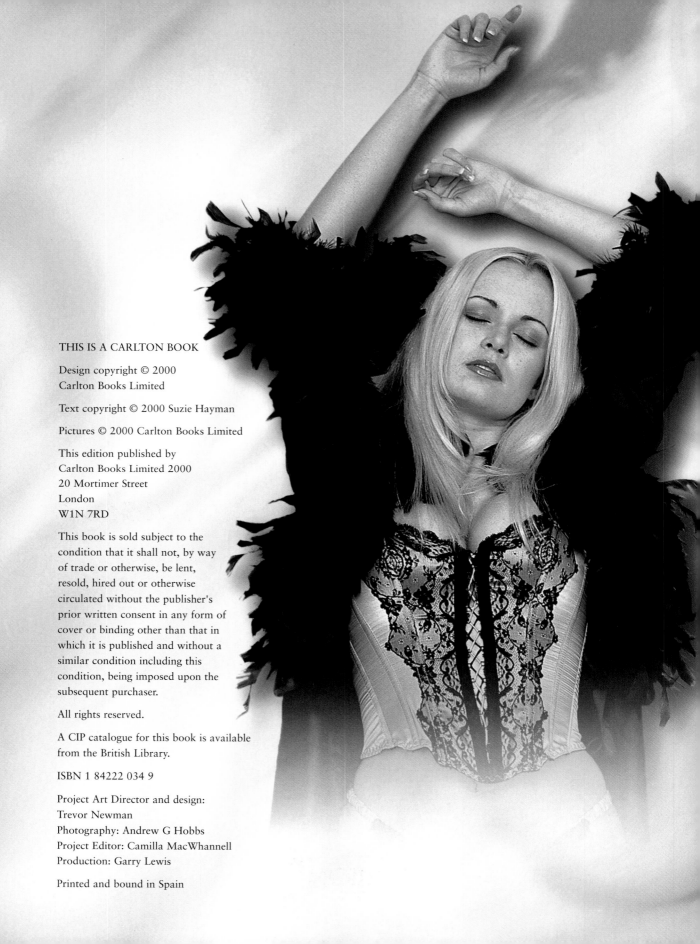

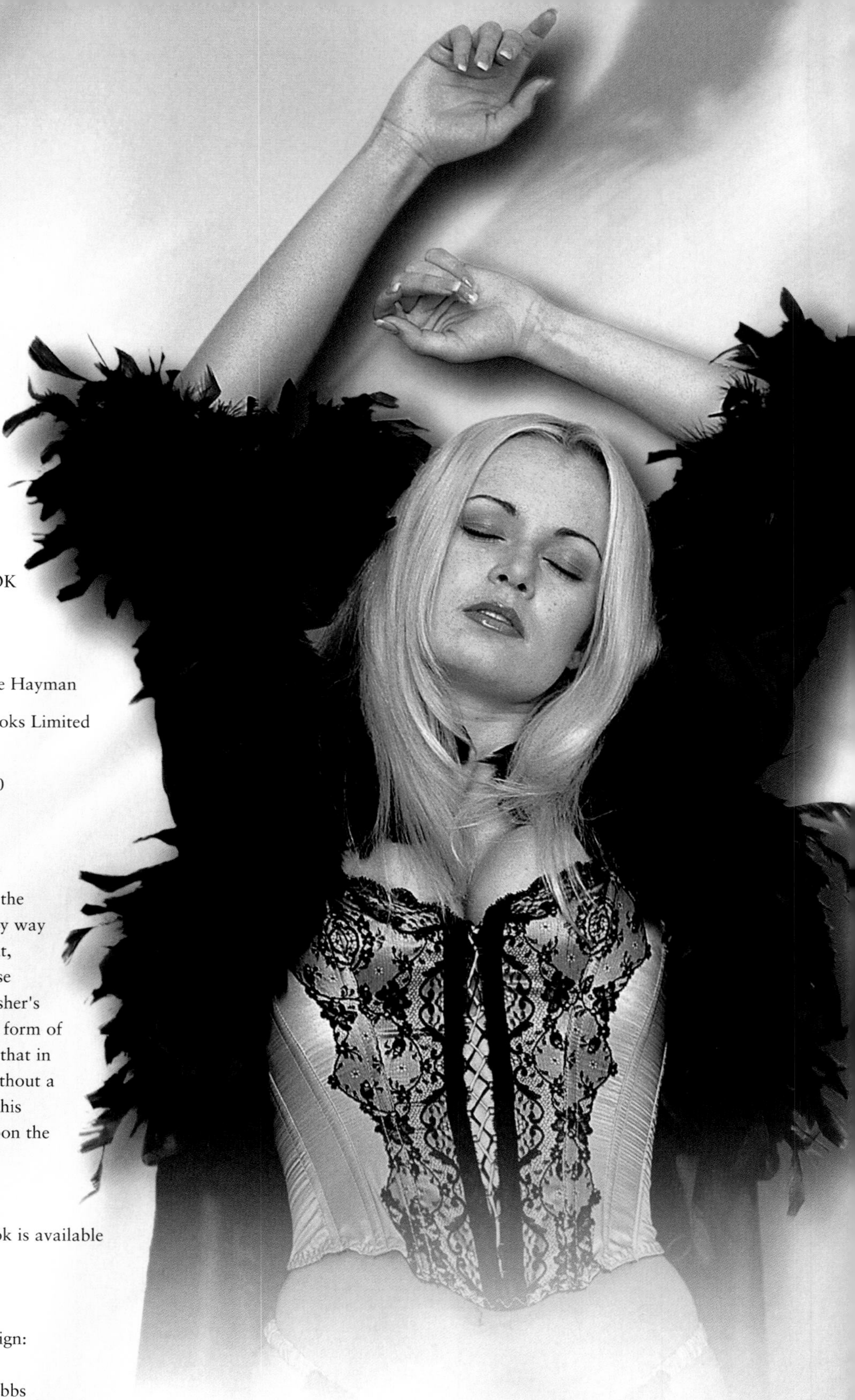

THIS IS A CARLTON BOOK

This edition published by
Carlton Books Limited 2000
20 Mortimer Street
London
W1N 7RD

A CIP catalogue for this book is available from the British Library.

ISBN 1 84222 034 9

Project Art Director and design:
Trevor Newman
Photography: Andrew G Hobbs
Project Editor: Camilla MacWhannell
Production: Garry Lewis

Printed and bound in Spain

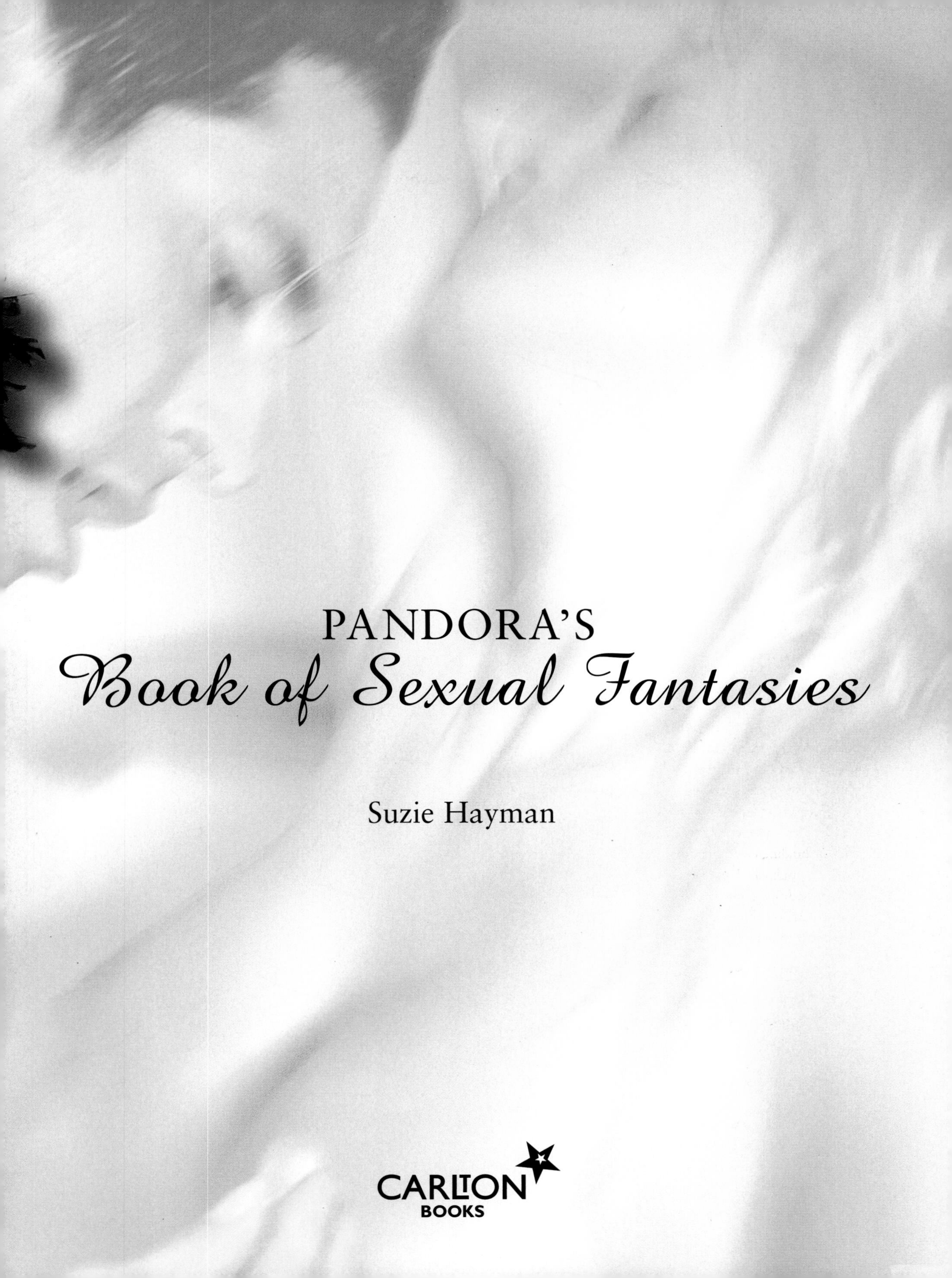

PANDORA'S
Book of Sexual Fantasies

Suzie Hayman

CARLTON BOOKS

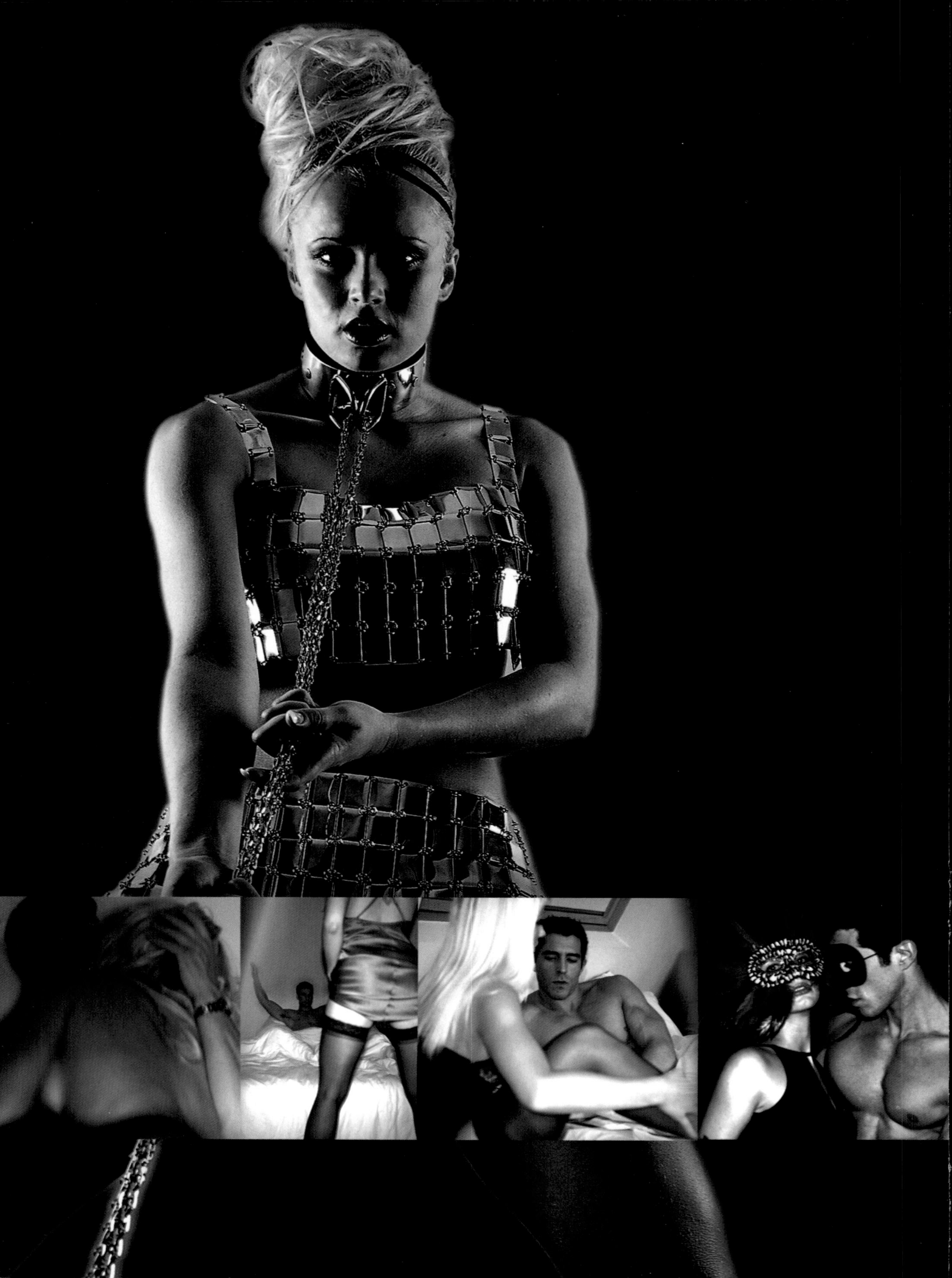

Contents

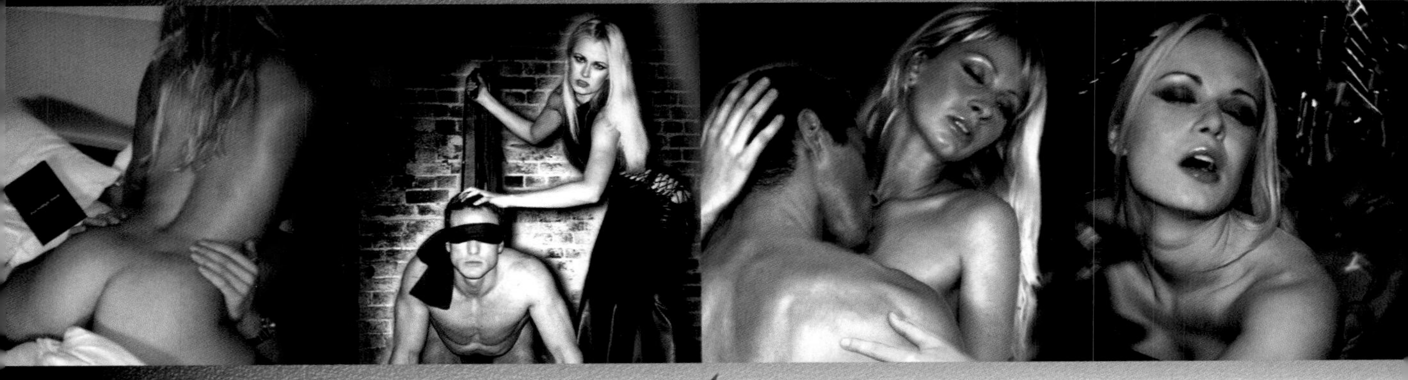

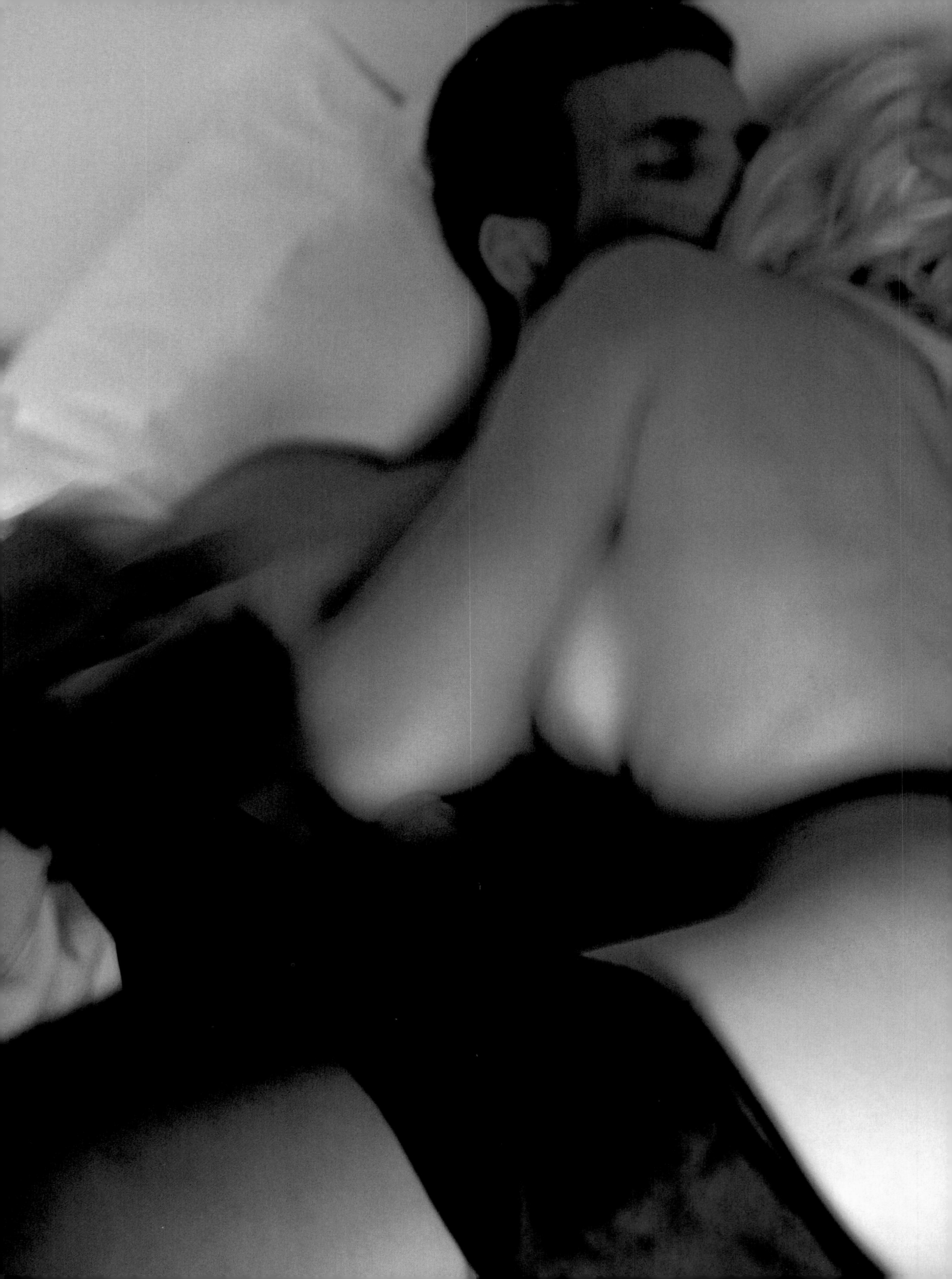

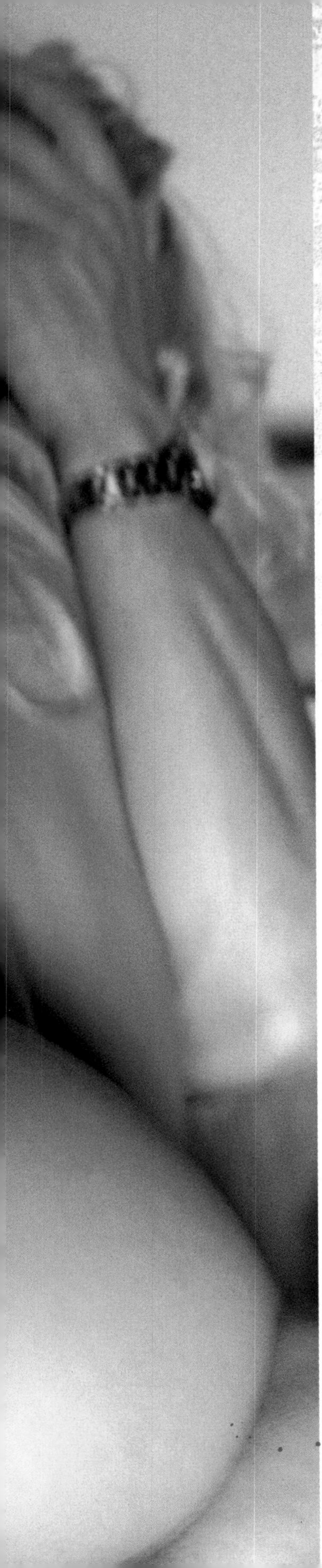

Sex should be fun. Of course we have sex for the serious business of having babies and furthering the species, but the fact is that on most of the occasions we make love pregnancy is the furthest thing from our minds.

INTRODUCTION

Sex should be fun. Of course we have sex for the serious business of having babies and furthering the species, but the fact is that on most of the occasions we make love pregnancy is the furthest thing from our minds.

You make love to express your feelings for your partner and to enjoy yourselves. It doesn't trivialize sex to acknowledge that, more times than not, pleasure and delight, fun and games, are the main driving forces. But there are two barriers to sexual bliss. One is lack of knowledge; knowledge about sex in general and knowledge about what turns you and your partner on in particular. The other is shyness and embarrassment. This produces a wariness that causes us to hold back from doing the things we'd really like to do with our partners. This is where we come in.

This book will be your gateway to a new sexual world together. Your new world will be one in which you can, and will, share knowledge and become more confident, more knowing and far more sensually and sexually accomplished. Most of us long for passion and romance. We want flirtation and fantasy, moonlight and roses. We want a relationship that has infatuation and excitement, lust and desire. We want to be endlessly surprised, to be thrilled and stimulated, both in and out of bed. We'd love to throw caution to the winds and fling ourselves into sexual adventures. We often don't, because we worry what the neighbours will think, or are scared our partners may be shocked. Or, more often, we simply don't know where to start. We need permission to give something different a go, we need to know that what we'd like is normal and acceptable. And we'd probably appreciate a few hints on what we could try.

This book is here to give you all that, and more. Turn the pages and set free a dazzling array of delicious ideas for any couple wanting to embark on new sexual adventures. You could be new lovers standing on the edge of a fresh love affair wondering how far to jump in to satisfy yourselves and your new partner. You could be an established couple in a sexual relationship of months, years or decades standing who are looking for new tricks for old dogs. Whether you're new or familiar, novice or experienced, young or old, straight or gay, you will find what you are looking for to put a kick in your love life.

Sharing a book at bedtime can be a prelude to more than just sleep

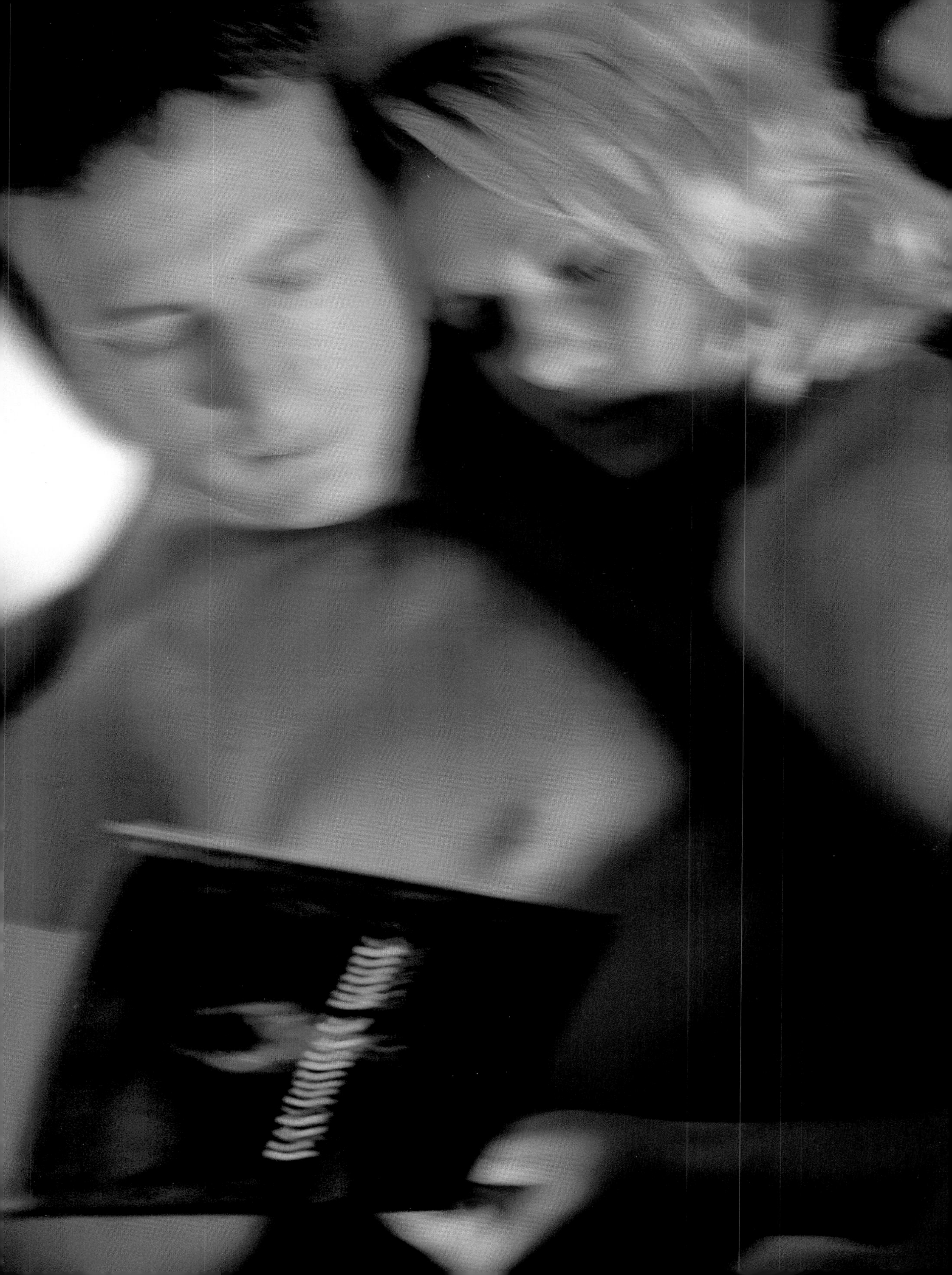

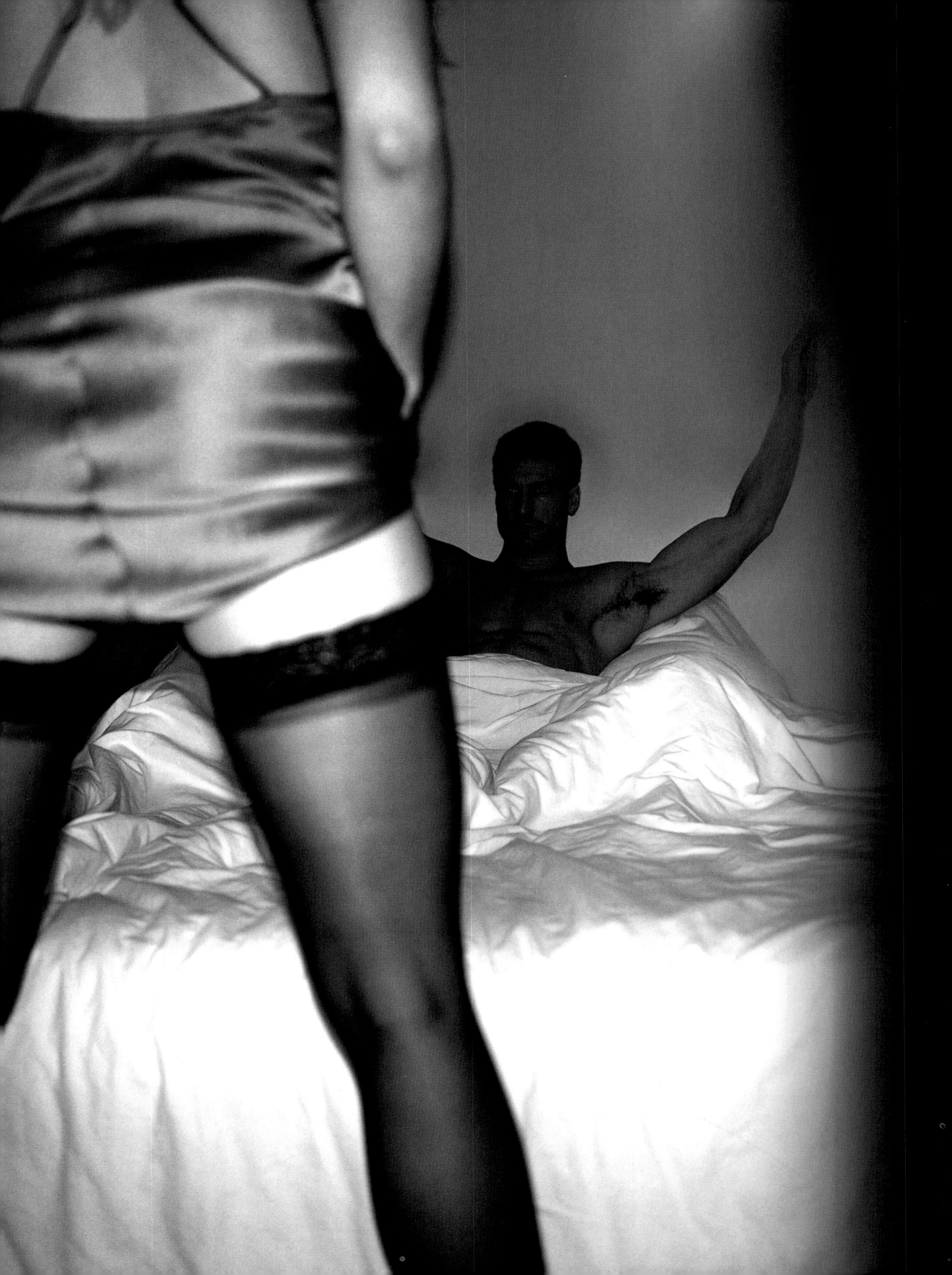

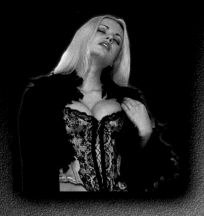

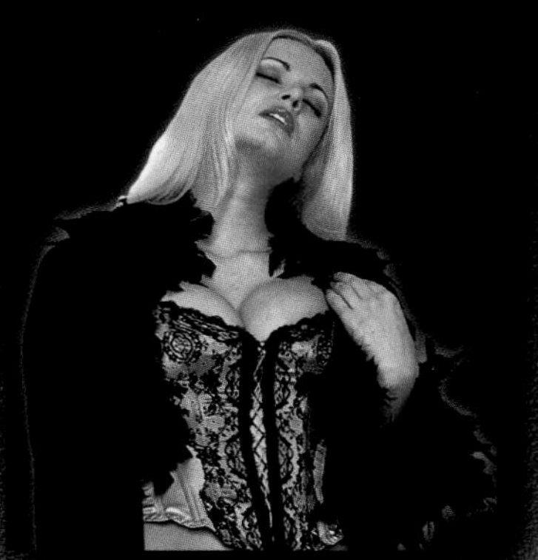

Chapter 1

THE FIRST STEPS TOWARDS SEXUAL ADVENTURES

Anyone can be a sexual adventurer – a pioneer of the bedroom, a trail-blazer, an explorer and a practitioner of the arts of the boudoir. We tend to think that the truly great lovers are people like Catherine of Russia or Don Juan; people who honed their flawless sexual technique with dozens of sexual partners. But being a good lover isn't about gargantuan sexual appetites and extensive lists of lovers. It isn't quantity but quality that makes you the lover your partner would choose above all others. You can have lots of notches on your bedpost and actually be terrible in bed if you assume that what works for one person at one time will always be sufficient or will have the same effect on anyone else.

You can be the lover you've dreamed of being, and have the love affair to rival Anthony and Cleopatra, Romeo and Juliet, Cathy and Heathcliffe (but without the tragic endings), with just a little imagination and a little practice. There are two keys to sexual ecstasy, in knowing how to please yourself and set your partner on fire. One is knowing yourself. The other is being able to keep an open mind and to be sensitive to your partner's responses. Sex isn't something that you learn how to do in one night, on one sexual encounter. It's a perpetual journey of discovery where you can constantly learn new things and explore new places. Let this book be your map and your guide, and your encouragement to start and keep travelling. The sensual starting point for every lover is self-knowledge. You're not born knowing how to arouse and satisfy yourself, let alone how to arouse or satisfy a sexual partner. The only way you're going to learn how is to find out for yourself, beginning by learning to please yourself. You don't have to understand the ins and outs of physiology to enjoy sex. Many people who write to me on my agony page worry about what they should be doing in bed to their partner, and what their partner should be doing to them. They ask for the definitive word on how to achieve sexual pleasure. If he twiddles this or she twitches that, if both fiddle about with the other, will it result in rapture? The answer has to be, "Well, sometimes, it depends." Because the real answer is that we're all different and what pleases you, or an ex-partner, may not be what pleases the next person. The path to true sexual pleasure, as well as the path to true love, is one you have to travel for yourselves. But don't look on this as a chore, or as homework that takes hours of grinding drudgery. On the contrary, it's a sensual journey of self-discovery, through scenery you'll delight in and toward a destination you'll enjoy once you arrive. You don't need to be told what should work for you; when it comes to sexual pleasure, we are all our own best experts. What you do need, however, is ideas to start with and the reassurance that it's OK to experiment. Most of us are surprisingly creative in our love lives if left alone to give it a go together. It's social pressure that makes us feel that sex is a taboo, no-go area, and spoils it for many couples. What can set you free is communication. If you can be open with your partner about what you feel, what you need and what you'd like (and your partner can talk to you too) you can be much more intimate and your sex life will rise to a different plane. In fact, sexual experts are fond of saying that only ten per cent of sexual excitement and pleasure is due to what we do with our bodies. The rest is down to what goes on in our minds – our expectation and anticipation, our emotions and imagination. Sex is mostly in the mind, so developing this powerful tool in terms of sharing fantasies and role-plays opens up a world of sexual endeavour that can make a couple's relationship dynamic and exciting. What this book will help you do is expand the potent force that is each individual's fantasy life, and help you bring this out to enhance your sexual relationship.

FROM CANDLES TO NIPPLE RINGS

Sexual adventuring can take many forms. It can range from lighting a few candles and dimming the lights to piercing your nipples, squeezing into a rubber suit, decking yourself out with chains and wielding a specially made riding crop. You don't have to try anything over the top, but lots of people do and it's neither unusual, abnormal nor strange to have a try at something new. To set your love life on fire and discover the ways you and your lover can really satisfy each other, you need to open up to your partner. But how far to go is the usual dilemma. The fear of so many couples is that if they told their partner what they'd really, really like, they're either going to recoil in horror, reel back in disgust or fall about laughing. Most lovers want to capture the imagination of their partner. You hope that your sexual relationship will be

The path to true sexual pleasure, as well as the path to true love, is one you have to travel for yourselves.

Right: Communication is vital in ensuring a couple's relationship is as fulfilling as possible

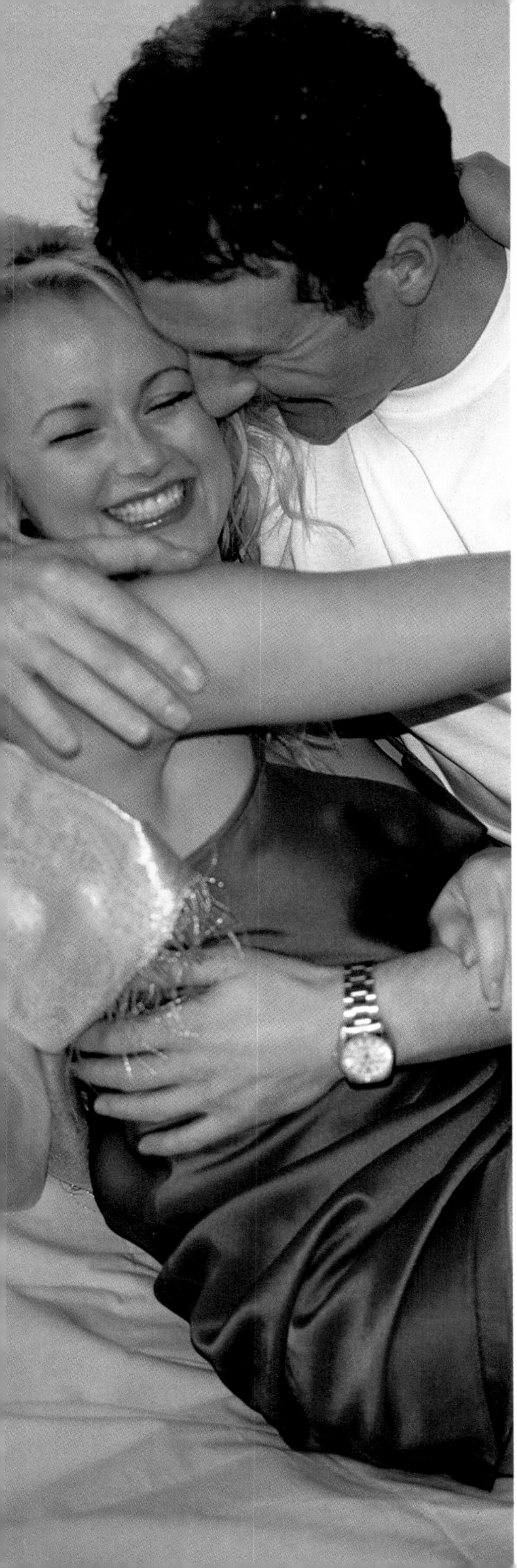

all-consuming and totally satisfying, for both of you. But how do you begin this journey of sexual exploration and enlightenment, how do you take the first steps to talk to each other and open up? This book will help you on your way, give you the confidence to fulfil each other's dreams and desires and show you how to improve your loving communication.

Understanding how to set the scene for a sensual experience can give you the impetus to add variety to your sex life together. But it also opens you up to feeling able to discuss your needs and desires, your fears and worries. We will lead you, step by step, to unleashing the full power of your sexual and sensual imagination. You'll be surprised how inventive and downright extravagant you can be, once you know such behaviour is allowed and even encouraged between lovers. One after the other, our scenarios will show you what is possible for lovers who would like to share a rich tapestry of new sexual ideas. You might think that the limit of what you can do in your love life is to slap on a bit of massage oil, lower the lights and maybe, just maybe, go crazy with a new sexual position or two. Soon, however, the sky will be your limit, with exciting games and experiences for you both to pursue.

Sexual adventure, as we've suggested already, begins with self-knowledge. The more confident you are in knowing your own unique repertoire of sexual responses and feelings, the easier it becomes to share this knowledge with your lover. The sad fact is that sex isn't always fun for everyone. Many people have difficulties in relationships, but a surprisingly high number of us, even when the love bit is going fine, find the sex bit leaves a lot to be desired. There are quite a few reasons for this. One of them is that we simply have neither the knowledge nor the practice to know how a partner can best satisfy us or we can please them. The urge to have sex may be instinctive, but realizing how to get the best out of it is not. As an agony aunt I get a lot of letters from women and men asking me how to have satisfying sex. The belief is that if I can tell them exactly what bits to push and pull in what particular order, satisfaction will be guaranteed. The reason why so many people have problems in the first place is that there is no "right" or "wrong" way of making love. I can tell you plenty of things to try. I can make loads of suggestions on what could be arousing and satisfying. I can give you literally hundreds of ideas of what lots of people find works for them. But you and your partner will have to find out for yourselves which ones really turn you on and work for you. This is why the very best advice anyone can give is "try it for yourself".

TAUGHT TO BE SHY

Now, we have a major problem with this. Little boys and little girls know instinctively that "try it for yourself" is an excellent way to get started and they tend to do so with a will almost from birth. Babies will explore their own bodies and so will toddlers. What they are doing is learning the limits of their own universe and recognizing where they stop and the rest of the world begins. But they are also finding, to joyous effect, just how good touching, pulling and tweaking feels. Then the snake enters their Eden. This is where most of us begin to have problems. Some parents will leave you to get on with your explorations, only gently persuading you, when a bit older, to keep it private so as not to offend others. But in the vast majority of cases we get our hands slapped. Sadly, this doesn't teach us that we shouldn't bring a blush to other people's faces. What it teaches us is that our bodies are dirty, our desires perverted and that sexual exploration is a thoroughly bad thing. Left to themselves, children make these discoveries as pre-schoolers and then put them away for future reference when they move on to that exciting time in their lives when they meet other people their own age, enter the fascinating world of school and the wide world and start to develop social skills. Several years later along comes puberty, the body awakens and all those lessons should be recalled and come into focus. As teenagers, most young people would then resume their happy exploration of their own body, gradually doing it in the company of another young person and the two of them benefiting from the lessons each have learned. Unfortunately, however, what generally happens is that when our hormones start telling us that the time is ripe what comes to the fore is our guilt and fear. Boys masturbate but do so hurriedly and furtively in order not to be caught out. What this gives them is an excellent grounding in premature ejaculation. Girls may masturbate, but if they do so know the lessons they are teaching themselves are not to be passed on to their partners. They know that if they tell a boy that they know how to bring themselves to orgasm, and try and show how he can do this for them, they are likely to get a very bad reputation indeed. Just as often, girls learn not to touch themselves at all. So it's hardly surprising when it comes to mutual lovemaking that they don't know how to give themselves pleasure and neither does their partner.

The more confident you are in knowing your own unique repertoire of sexual responses and feelings, the easier it becomes to share this knowledge with your lover.

But there's no reason to despair since it's never too late to catch up. If you haven't learned your lessons while young, or they are shrouded in confusion, fear and guilt, the answer is to catch up now at whatever stage you are in your life. Self-exploration and self-understanding is the key to good lovemaking in a relationship. Don't believe the myth that masturbation is for losers or will spoil you for the real thing. An orgasm is an orgasm, however you reach it: by yourself, by your own actions but with your partner present, by your partner's caresses or through your dreams and fantasies. What you learn on your own you can pass on to your partner to your mutual benefit and joy.

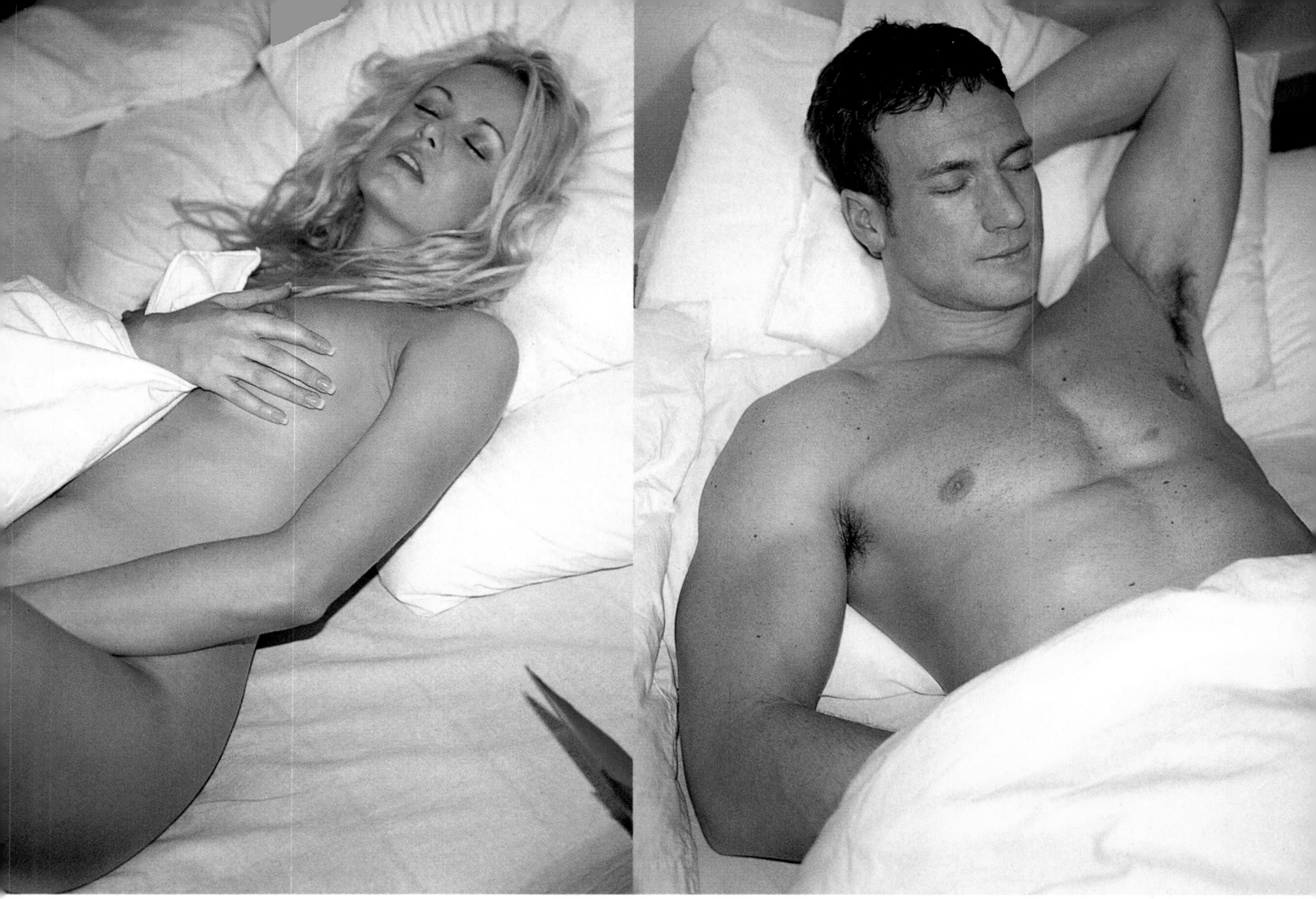

Self-exploration and self-understanding is the key to good lovemaking in a relationship

HOW TO APPRECIATE YOURSELF

Start your new journey to marvellous sex by learning how to appreciate yourself. It's hard for anyone either to accept or give sexual pleasure if they don't like themselves. One of the sad results of being made to feel that sensual exploration is bad is not only to tell you that your sexual desires are unacceptable but that you are too. Children who have been made to feel that they shouldn't be touching themselves often come out of childhood with a feeling that not only are their desires wrong but their body is too. They have a subtle sense of overall "wrongness" that is often expressed in fears that their bodies are ugly or deformed. Doctors, counsellors and agony aunts often hear from people convinced that their bodies are saggy, lumpy, wrinkled and covered in ugly and unusual stretch-marks; that they are deformed, too fat, too thin, too tall, too short; that their genitals are the wrong shape, the wrong size, the wrong colour or texture; that they smell, are far too hairy or not hairy enough. What is invariably held up for disgusted examination is a perfectly normal, perfectly acceptable body. So, strip off, stand in

What you learn on your own you can pass on to your partner to your mutual benefit and joy.

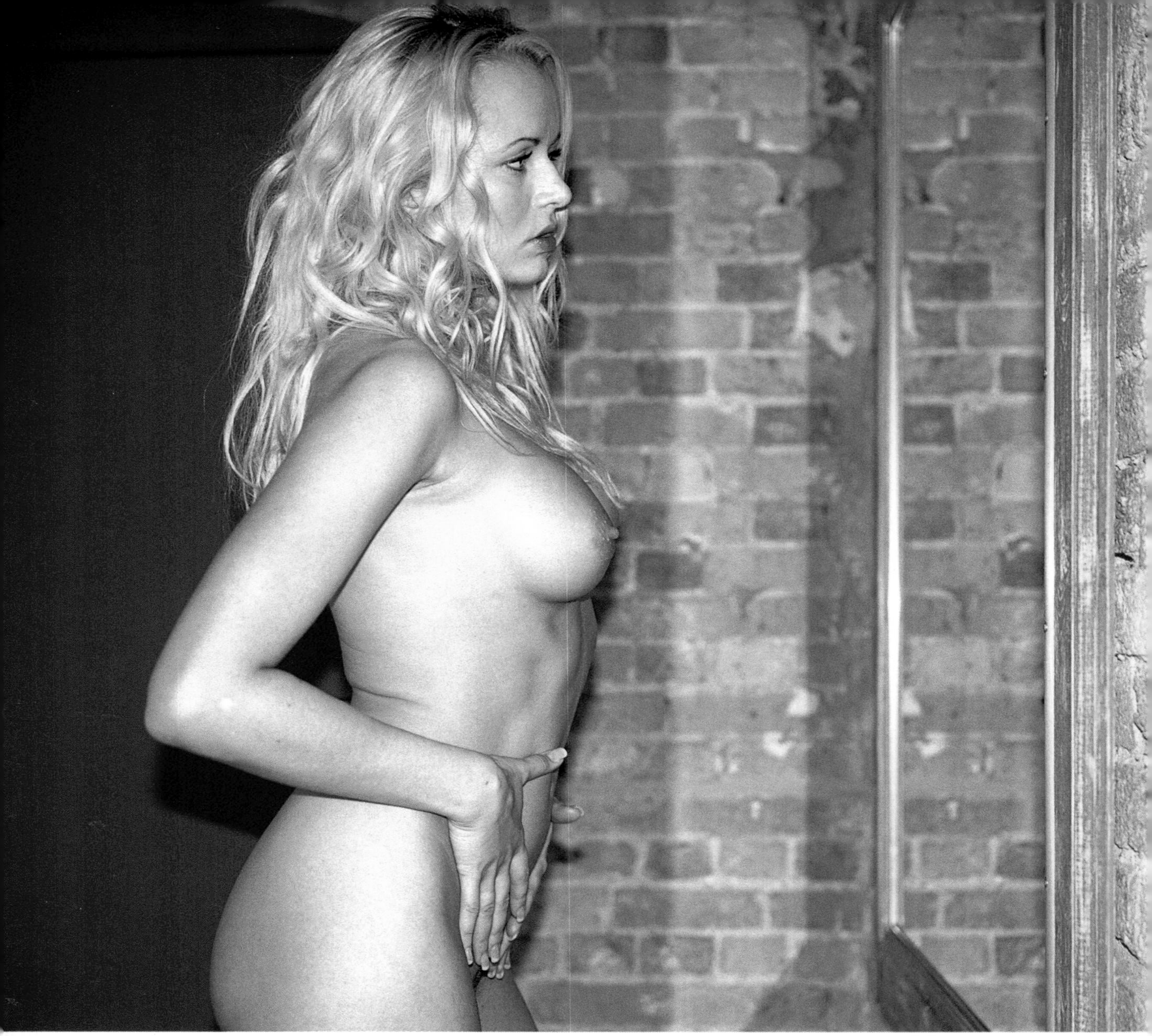

Learn to appreciate yourself. Strip off, stand in front of a mirror and look at yourself

front of a mirror and look at yourself. Slowly scrutinize yourself from top to bottom, side to side and all the way round. What do you see? Fat thighs, ugly genitals – too small if you are a guy, too hairy if you are a woman? If you are a woman do you think your breasts are too big, too small, too droopy or have too many stretch-marks? If you are a man do you think you haven't enough muscles or enough hair – or too much? How does your body make you feel? Disgusted, despairing, depressed or angry?

Now have another look at yourself. When you make those negative judgements, whose voice do you hear saying those things? Is it a parent, school-mates, a previous or present partner? If it's your own voice, who or what is really behind the judgement? Can you hear any positive sounds, voices that tell you what lovely skin texture you have, what a gorgeous neck, what lovely breasts or balls you have? Take another look and consider what someone who loved you would see with fresh eyes. All those standards that say you have to be slimmer or not as thin, better endowed or neater, hairier or less hairy –

Once you've sensitized yourself and brought yourself alive by stroking yourself, you can concentrate on finding the next level.

who really sets them and why? You are beautiful, whatever your shape or size, and the sooner you realize that, the better for you, your partner and your love life. Look at yourself and pick one bit of yourself that you like, and tell yourself, "You have beautiful eyes/nipples/hair." Say it again, and promise that you'll tell yourself this again at least once a day. Each day, find another part of you that you realize is attractive, and add it to the litany. Ask your partner which parts they find attractive, and look at that part of your body with a new appreciation.

So now close your eyes and slowly and carefully run your hands all over your body, gently feeling and experiencing yourself. How does it feel to have your hands glide over your body, and what sensations do you have from your hands when they touch your body? Are you wincing, giggling or feeling ticklish? Do you feel shy or awkward? Are those voices now saying that feeling pleasure is bad, naughty, not for you because you don't deserve it? Imagine taking all those negative messages, wrapping them up in a parcel and putting them where they belong – back in the hands of the person who made them. Let them deal with them! Or, you can imagine putting them in the dustbin, with the trash, where they belong. Now you've got rid of all that sad baggage that has held you back, move on. Now run your hands over yourself again and concentrate and begin to see how very pleasant you feel. Notice the different textures there are to skin, depending on whether it's skin on your face or the back of your hands, the soles of your feet or the inside of your thighs that you're touching. Focus on the palms of your hands – are they rough and callused or soft and smooth, and which texture would feel better on which parts of your body? Feel the hair on your body – is it really too much or too little, or is the texture delightful to feel, just like a warm and cuddly animal?

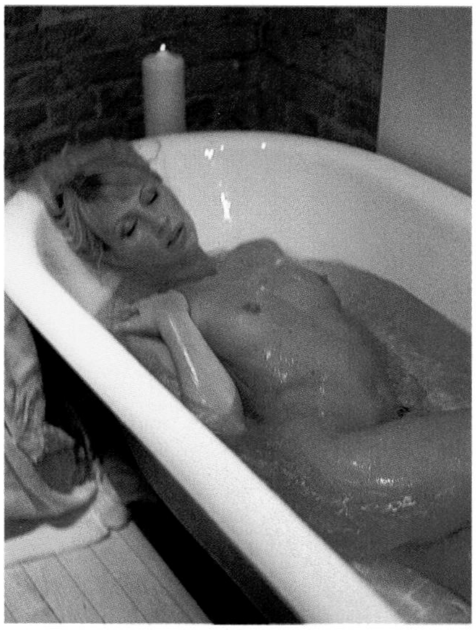

Explore simple and usual pleasures in a warm bath

FOCUSED EXPLORATION

Now it's time to move on to some more focused exploration. For this you might like to sit or lie down. Make sure you are warm and comfortable. It helps, for instance, to have some cream or oil on hand or even to do this in a warm bath with plenty of bath oil or gel in the water. Again, run your hands slowly over yourself from top to bottom, side to side and all around. This time concentrate on what seems especially pleasant. You are looking for three levels of enjoyment. The first is the simple, animalistic, sensual pleasure of being touched. All of us, whether we are cats or humans, love the power of touch. There is nothing quite as comforting and valuing as being stroked. Pass your hands over the fur of a cat and it will purr. Try it on yourself and allow yourself to see why the animal makes that noise. Focus, and you'll soon find that when you can get beyond the messages that tell you to disapprove of self-pleasure, there isn't a part of your body that you can't appreciate being touched.

Once you've sensitized yourself and brought yourself alive by stroking yourself, you can concentrate on

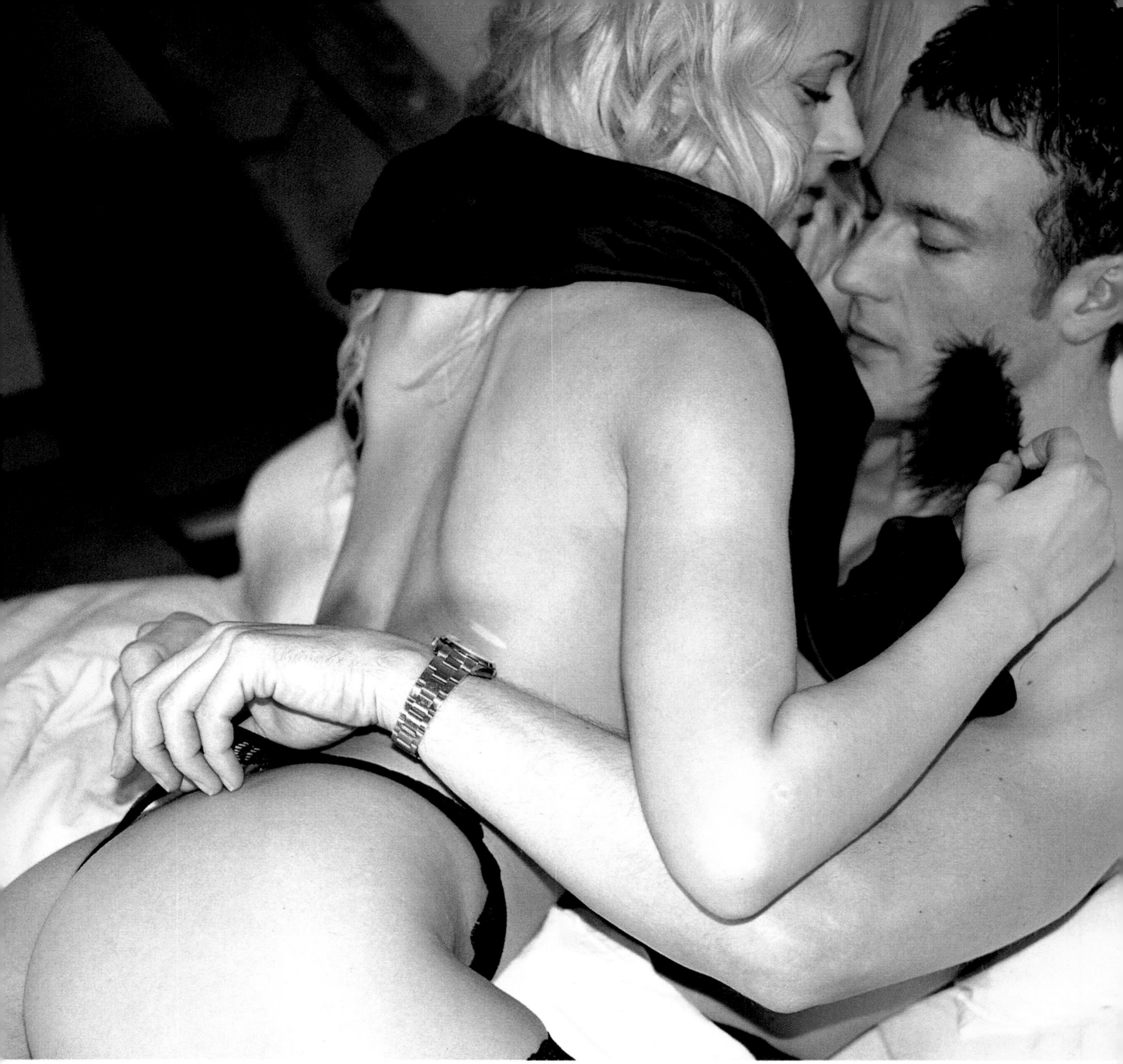

Most parts of the body respond to stimulation. It's fun to find out together what feels good

finding the next level. This is to find and bring to life the parts of your body that tingle not only with sensual pleasure but which respond with sexual arousal to your caresses. There are obvious places – the nipples of both sexes, the clitoris and the penis. Perhaps you won't be surprised to discover that the lips are also intensely sensitive, and most of us know that earlobes react strongly enough to have you sexually excited when they are stimulated. You wouldn't be amazed to find that the labia and the scrotum are intensely sensitive or that sucking, blowing on or nibbling toes and fingers is likely to get a good response. Most people notice their necks are extremely sensitive as are the inside of the elbows and thighs and the backs of the knees. But what about the buttocks or small of the back, around the anus, down the inside of the thighs? How do you react to having your back stroked or the tops of your feet tickled? You may also find the way you stimulate a particular part of the body has a bearing on the way it may or may not arouse you. Stroke and touch and experiment with different levels of touching to see what sort of effect they have. You can brush lightly with the tips or flats of your fingers or scratch gently with your nails. You can tickle or rub lightly or more firmly. You can use the heels of your hands to massage rhythmically or press and knead with your thumbs. You can use the palms or the whole of your hand to stroke or brush large areas of your body or concentrate on just one bit. Find those parts of yourself that particularly bring you to shivering pleasure when stimulated. Experiment with the various caresses that can really get you going.

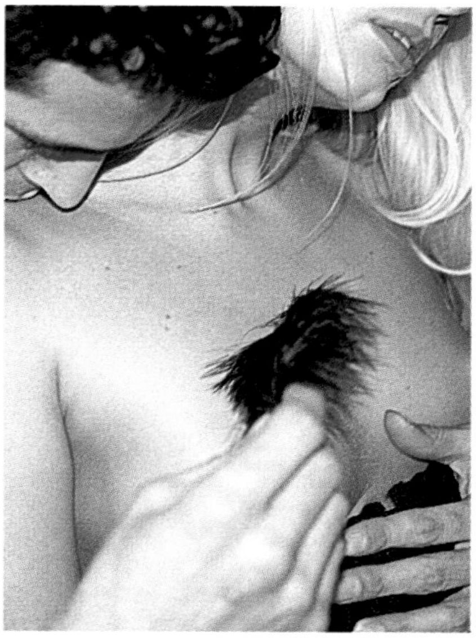

Use a feather to tease and tweak and touch

PLEASE YOURSELF

When you've found what sets you up, it's time to move on to discovering how you can really please yourself, from arousal to full satisfaction. Concentrate on those areas that particularly excite you, but try not to stimulate only the most obvious bits. You can predictably bring yourself to an orgasm by rousing your penis or clitoris, but both your arousal and climax will be more exciting and satisfying if you stimulate as much as your body as possible rather than just going for the main act. Take your time and imagine you're painting – a detailed portrait or a massive landscape. Use your fingers and anything else that comes to hand to build up layers of sensation and reaction. Self-pleasuring can be all the more satisfying if you introduce different ways of fondling yourself – strokes, caresses, nips, pinches, scratches and even smacks – but also if you introduce contrasting textures. Pour some oil or cream on yourself and see how it feels to glide and squidge your hands all over your body. Use a feather to tease and tweak and touch. Use some fake fur, a silk scarf or a scratchy facecloth or towel. See the difference if you dip a sponge first into hot water and then into cold before wiping it over the sensitive parts of your body. There is no rush, so pursue every last scrap of enjoyment. Pay especial attention to anything that seems to set your teeth on edge or make you jump – pain or discomfort is often the other side of the coin to pleasure. So if at first it makes you shy away it could in fact be the touch that is going to give you the greatest result. Bring yourself to full arousal and continue until you've come to an orgasm. And you need not stop

Take your time and imagine you're painting – a detailed portrait or a massive landscape. Use your fingers and anything else that comes to hand to build up layers of sensation and reaction.

there. Both sexes find being hugged and held particularly comforting after orgasm, so hug yourself to complete the pleasure. You are likely to enjoy the sensation of rhythmic stroking on your arms, face and back for some time after orgasm. For some people, it need not stop with the first orgasm. The vast majority of women are capable of several orgasms at a time. Continue to explore your sensations after you have come and you may find the next climax is even better than the last. Some men can also discover a potential for multi-orgasms – you will only find out if you are multi-orgasmic if you try it.

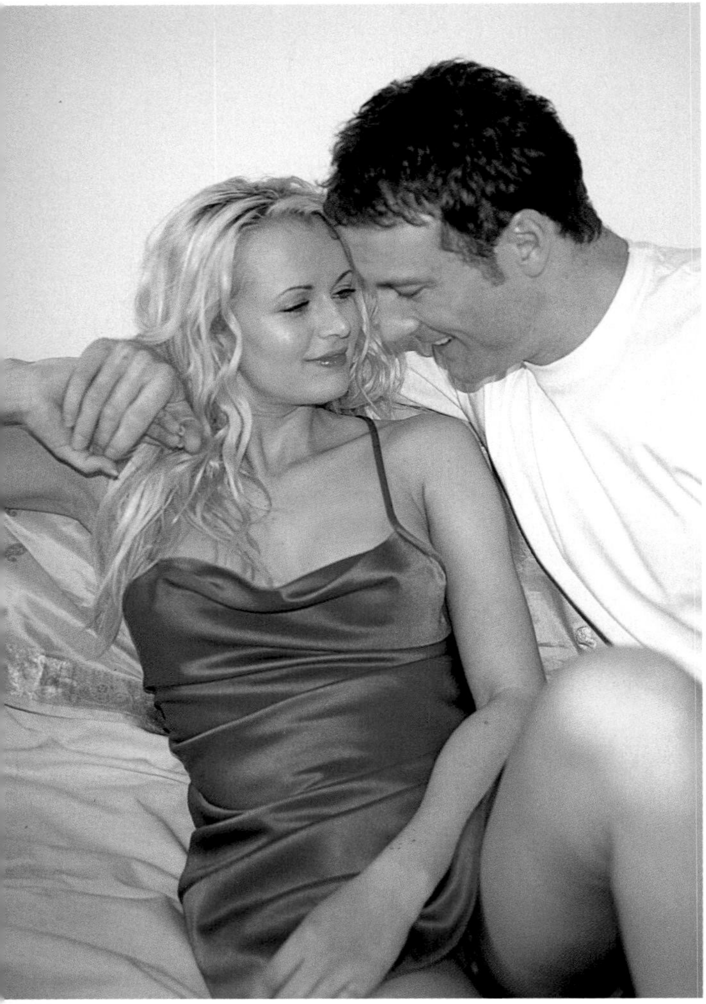

The key is communication.

You can make these discoveries on your own or try them in the presence of your partner. Whatever, you are likely to learn the most if you each let your fingers do the walking on yourselves first. Once you've gained some confidence and experience in what feels good to you it's time to move on to sharing this with your partner. Settle down in comfort and privacy with them. Agree beforehand that you'll begin with a show-and-tell session, with each of you promising to watch, listen and learn. Take turns demonstrating what you've found to your partner. Touch your own body, talking your partner through how various caresses feel in different places. Bring yourself to arousal and then to climax as your partner watches. You could do this simultaneously, but what often happens then is that you get caught up in your own sensations and forget to notice what is going on with your partner. Do this together a few times before moving on to the next stage, which is where you each put what you've learned from each other into practice. Snuggle up together and start showing how well you've understood your lessons.

Touch your own body, talking your partner through how various caresses feel in different places.

COMMUNICATION – THE BEST FORM OF ORAL SEX

The key is communication. Of course communication comes in several ways. You can let your partner know what you are thinking and feeling by telling them. This isn't always easy. Along with being told that our bodies are "not quite nice" we are also told from an early age that sex talk is dirty. We tend to have three sets of vocabulary to describe sexual behaviour, sexual feelings and sexual parts of the body. One of them is the clinical, the other is obscene and the third is coy and euphemistic. So when you start to make love to a partner there is quite a dilemma. Do you call what you are doing "having intercourse", "shagging" or

The longer you take to build up to the last act, the more you will enjoy not only the ending but also the getting there.

" going the whole way"? You may find the words jar and feel awkward or indeed you may find they are exciting in themselves. Talking dirty is often a surprisingly vivid boost to your sexual enjoyment so this is another area in which the two of you will need to explore, experiment and find your own way. Whatever, letting your partner know that if he touches this area or that if she does that, it's going to set off the fireworks is the path to sexual bliss. But words are not the only way to get the meaning over. If you can, let your partner know they are getting it right with a sigh, a gasp or by body movement. Saying "Mmmmmmmm!" or going loose and floppy gets the message across as meaningfully as saying "I say, when you do that to me it really has the desired effect." The only important thing to keep in mind is that your partner can't read your mind. If you want them to get it right – and believe it, your partner definitely wants to get it right – you are going to have to let them know. And, of course, they are going to have to let you know, so listening with your whole body as well as your ears is vitally important. If you're not sure, ask them and check it out.

As with the self-exploration, do take your time. There is a great temptation when we get up close and personal to rush straight on to the main bit of the act. When we talk about making love or having sex what usually comes to mind is full-on intercourse leading up to climax. It's what we think of as the point of erotic activity and it's often the only part we consider or value, which is a great pity. Go for a drive through the mountains and it's not only the stop on the peak that will have you oohing and aahing. The journey itself is just as important, just as pleasurable. And the fact is that the better and more prolonged the journey is, the more you'll enjoy the final flourish. You can see lovemaking in exactly the same frame. The longer you take to build up to the last act, the more you will enjoy not only the ending but also the getting there. So, just as you did for yourself, lie with your partner and each of you start by running your hands all over the other's body. As with yourself, use the tips and flats of your fingers, the palms and the whole of your hands and vary your strokes from feather touches, scratches and nips to kneads and light slaps. Feel and probe and tell each other how much pleasure you are getting from touching them and listen for what they can tell you about how they are receiving your ministrations. Once you have acquainted yourself with your partner's entire body and they have with yours, focus more intently on what arouses and stimulates each other. This is where you need to direct your partner to the parts of your body that respond especially and to let them do the same for

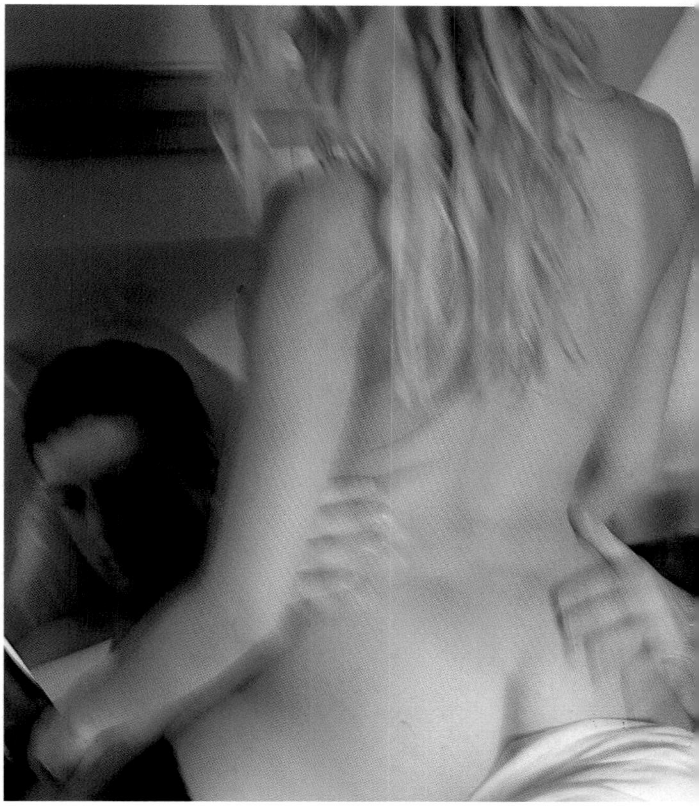

Help your partner to learn to please you

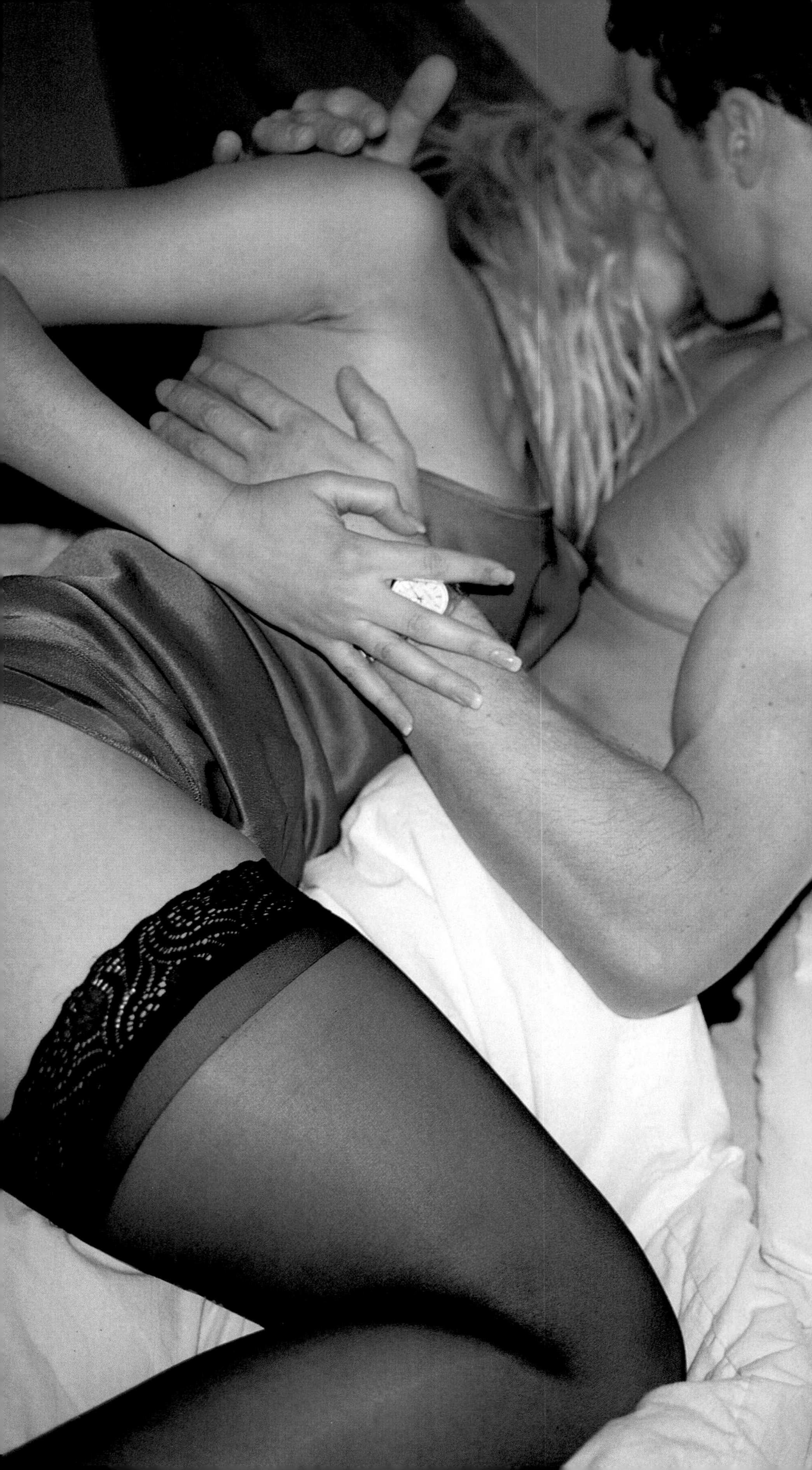
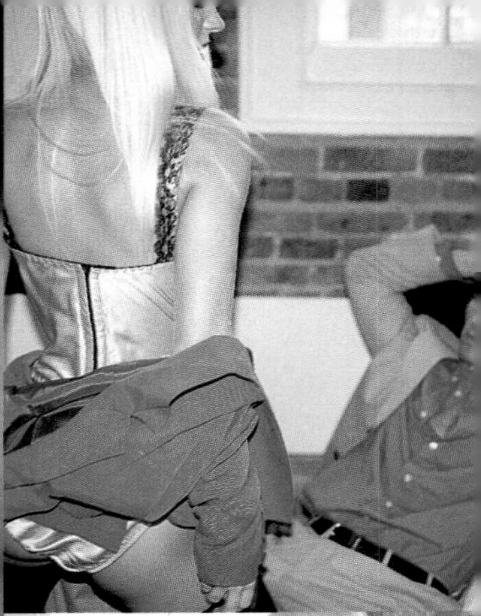
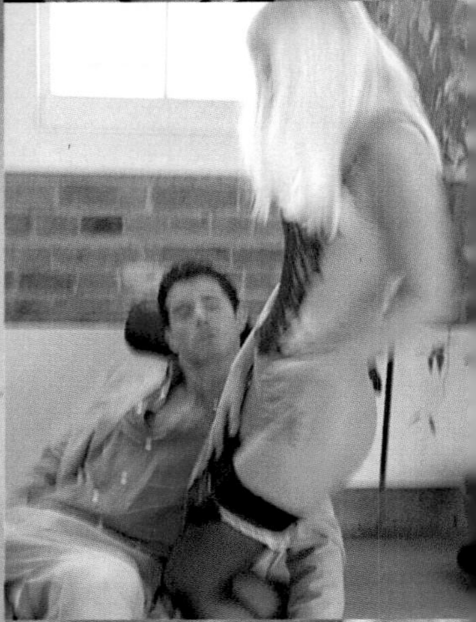
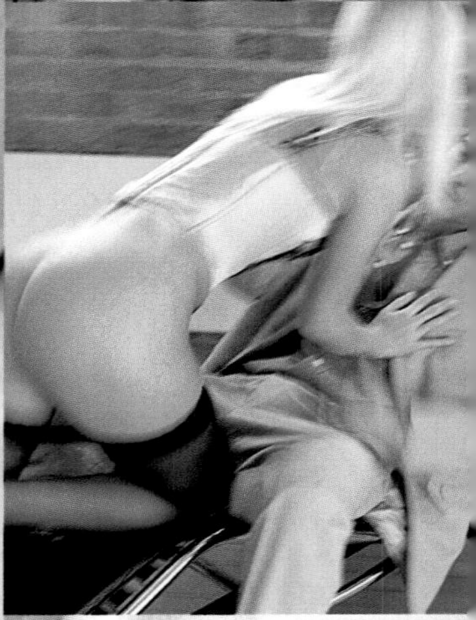
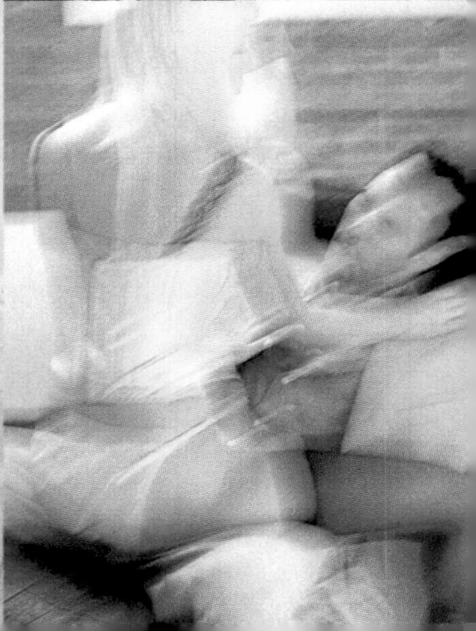

you. Keep in mind each other's individuality. What works for one of you may not for the other. In fact, what drives you wild might leave your partner cold or even irritated. Just because something may give you specific pleasure don't assume you should try it out on them or that they will like it. Let your partner help you to explore and learn what really pleases them and let them learn what pleases you. When you are both purring and relaxed you can really move on to focusing on turning up the flames of desire. Even at this point you should prolong the delicious agony. Just as too many lovers dash on into trying sexual arousal before they have fully explored sensual stimulation, so too do many people leap straight into penetrative sex before they've had time to explore the power of arousal without intercourse.

INTERCOURSE DOESN'T ALWAYS DO IT FOR WOMEN

The problem is that intercourse itself is highly pleasurable and extremely efficient at producing orgasms...for men! But there is an engineering problem when it comes to women. A man's climax is wonderfully and delightfully easily achieved simply by encasing his penis in the snug, warm embrace of a vagina. This has led many men to believe not only that their female partners will get the same result with the same method, but that an orgasm is best achieved by this means. For a woman to have an orgasm, however, she needs her clitoris to be stimulated, and this isn't always best done through intercourse. It is true that the network of nerves connected to the clitoris sweep back an extraordinary long way from that small organ sited above and in front of the urethra or water passage. The clitoris has been estimated as having an area of sensitivity some thirty times larger, size for size, than a penis. This means that even during vaginal penetration the movements in this area are transmitted to the clitoris, often leading to orgasm. But many women find more direct stimulation is necessary. They prefer either to have their clitoris touched directly by their own or their partner's fingers or for different sexual positions to allow stimulation in other ways. But in many cases, what makes a woman really enjoy sex is for there to be stimulation, direct and indirect, to the clitoris both before and after intercourse and for penetrative sex not to be the be-all and end-all of the act.

To get the full benefit of exploring and getting to know your own and your partner's body and reactions you could try this game. The first time you make love together ban penetrative sex altogether. Make the point of the exercise to see just how long you and your partner can go on enjoying your caresses and being aroused by what you are doing together without coming to a climax. Prolong your enjoyment for as long as possible. When you deny yourself the accustomed and quick and easy release of penetrative sex you will often find new ways of pleasing and being pleased. You may find that the pleasure you can give each other can certainly be longer, and may be better, when using hands, lips, tongues, feathers and anything else that comes to reach, instead of your genitals. Try it that way for several sessions before you bring in intercourse. You could go one step further and try "Look, Ma, no hands!" sex. With this, not only is penetrative sex

Let your partner help you to explore and learn what really pleases them and let them learn what pleases you. When you are both purring and relaxed you can really move on to focusing on turning up the flames of desire.

Explore the power of arousal before leaping headlong into having intercourse

Fantasies should be fun. There's nothing weird or unusual in having them or using them to enhance your love life.

banned, but so is using hands and fingers. You can use tongues, lips and teeth. You can use feathers, fur and ice cream, or anything else that takes your fancy just so long as you don't use your hands. By experimenting and using your ingenuity, you will make intercourse just one of many ways to please each other instead of the one and only.

ADDITIONS TO A GOOD SEX LIFE

But all this fun and games won't detract from the serious side of sex. Having fun in bed does not mean being irresponsible or taking vows or commitments lightly. Respect and care for your partner are vital and basic requirements for any relationship, whether it's a new one that might not last long or an old one that has stayed the course. If you can't laugh and enjoy sex and come away from lovemaking feeling better than when you started, what's the point? And there are so many ways you and your partner can liven up, expand and deepen your intimate life together. You can dress for sex so that you excite your lover with your appearance – and undress for sex in ways that drive them wild. Read on and you'll find a wealth of ideas on how you can use clothing and other body adornment to enhance your love life. You can add the use of sex toys into your sexual repertoire – creams and oils, vibrators and dildos, straps, feathers and dice. We take a tour through the wide variety available, with suggestions of what to use, how to use them and games you can play to get you started. As you develop your sexual confidence further, you can experiment with of all sorts of sexual positions and exotic sexual variations. There are supposed to be literally hundreds of positions you can adopt when making love – we set you off discovering some that you may not have imagined, let alone tried.

Above all, you can develop and take pleasure in your sexual fantasies, perhaps one of the most important and certainly the most common additions to our sex lives. We all have sexual fantasies. They may be thoughts and wishes that pop into our minds and play themselves out without any conscious control, or they may be full-blown sexual dramas that you make up deliberately and which proceed in your mind as you plan. When you have a sexual fantasy, you're using the largest sexual organ in your body: your brain. Knowing how to use it best is the key to a happy sex and love life. Fantasies should be fun. There's nothing weird or unusual in having them or using them to enhance your love life. Not only do most of us have sexual fantasies, most of us have similar ones. That isn't to say your dreams aren't unique. But it is to reassure you that you're neither strange nor odd in finding these thoughts and ideas exciting, sexually arousing and stimulating. When you have read the full array of ideas, you should feel ready and able to let rip with your partner and explore your own particular favourites. There are three ways you can make sexual fantasies work for you. Some people use sexual fantasies just in their heads. But others tell their partners what's on their minds and find this adds enormously to their love lives. Finally, plenty of couples act out their sexual fantasies, using their imaginations and play-acting skills to put zest into their lovemaking.

THE POWER OF SEXUAL FANTASIES

The important point to note about fantasies is that they aren't real. There are plenty of scenarios that give us a thrill in our imaginations that might – or most certainly should – leave a bad taste if they happened in actuality rather than just being acted out. The idea of having sex with a much younger person is one. In reality, seducing a youngster who is under age is sexual abuse. Two other very common fantasies that might surprise you are of being taken by force, and having sex with someone of the gender opposite to the one you usually have sex with. Straight people often fantasize about gay sex, gay people fantasize about straight sex. It doesn't actually mean they necessarily want to change their sexual orientation. The reason both of these are common is that having or enjoying a particular fantasy usually has no bearing on how

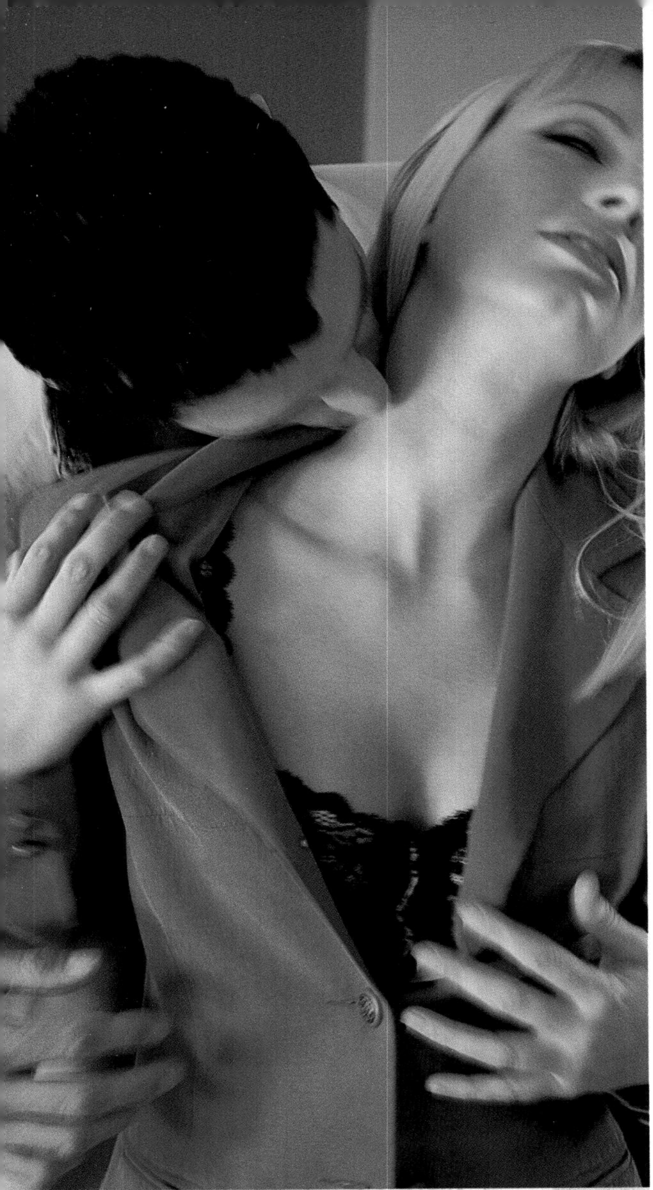

By reinventing yourselves and your relationship, just for a short time, you can take back to your partnership and your everyday relationship a whole new fresh perspective and some invigorating ideas.

we do, or would like to behave, in real life. You can dream about and play-act something while having absolutely no intention of doing it. In fact, half the thrill comes from that uneasy sense that what you're playing about with is unacceptable, to society as a whole or to you in particular, if you did it genuinely. This is why so many people find themselves drawn to sexual fantasies that seem so strange or worrying. A woman imagining having sex with another woman, a man with another man, or envisioning your partner having sex with you in spite of your saying no, are both very common sexual fantasies – from people who would not welcome a same-sex relationship, and would hate to be taken against their will. It's nothing to worry about if you find yourself having such fantasies and taking pleasure in them. Simply enjoying thoughts like these doesn't mean you want to put them into action. Of course, drawing the line and recognizing the boundaries is important. To be able to enjoy this book to full, glorious and satisfying effect, you and your partner should know the difference between fun and harm, love and abuse, mutual pleasure and exploitation.

SETTING THE SCENE

If you would like to act out your sexual fantasies with your partner, the key to doing so successfully and letting your imagination loose is to set the scene. You can, and should, improvise and be spontaneous. But feeling confident enough to throw your inhibitions away and immerse yourself in the play often depends on doing your homework first. If you can arrange the room and your props, have the story and some of your lines agreed and clear in your minds, you'll find it surprisingly easy to let rip and become different people, in a different place. With increased confidence and practice, you'll soon be making up your own scenarios and writing your own scripts. But if you're new to this, or have run through your own repertoire, we offer a smörgasbord of sexy ideas to try out. Above all, be reassured that sexual fantasies and imaginative sex play can do wonders for any relationship. By reinventing yourselves and your relationship, just for a short time, you can take back to your partnership and your everyday relationship a whole new fresh perspective and some invigorating ideas.

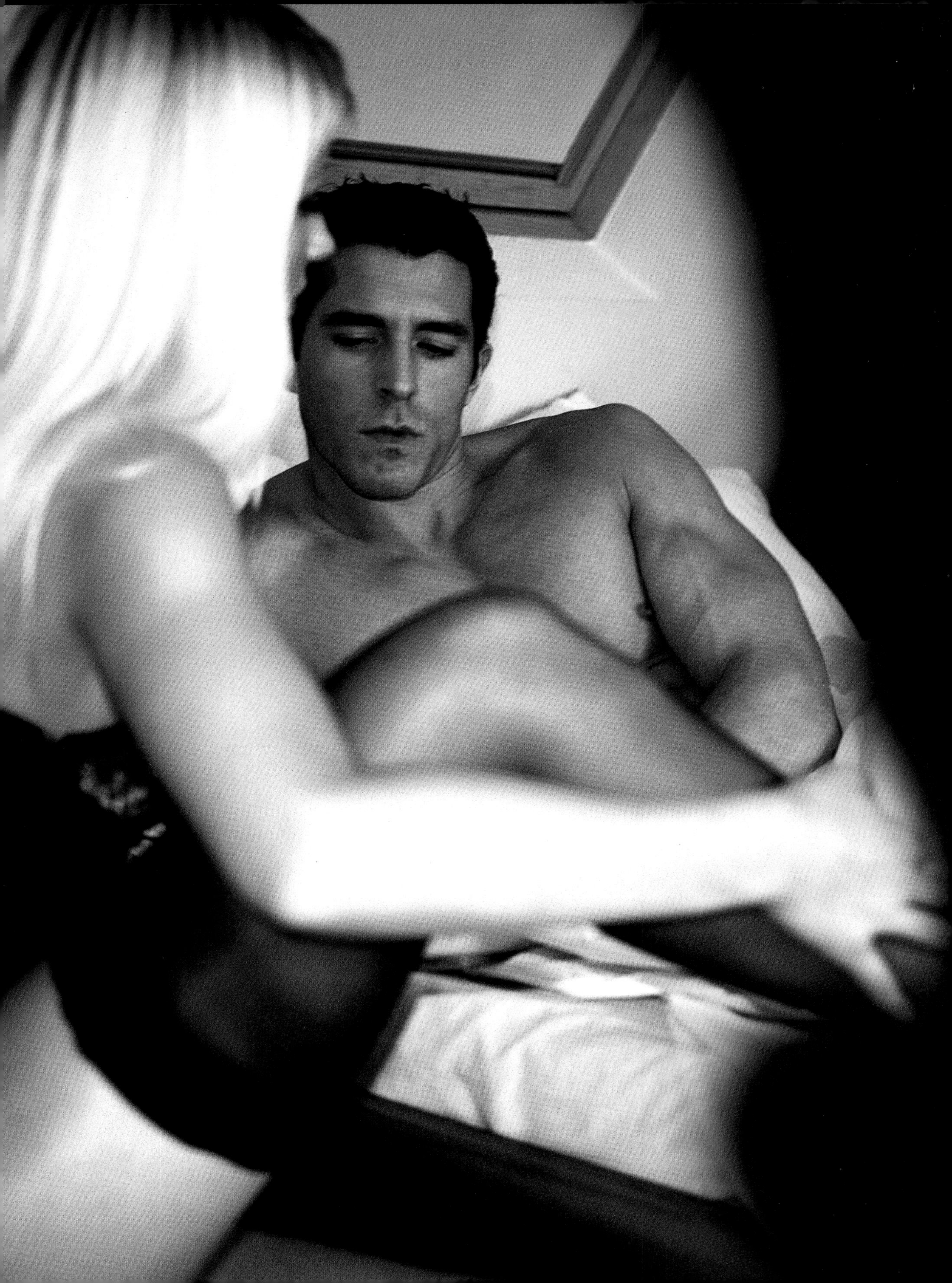

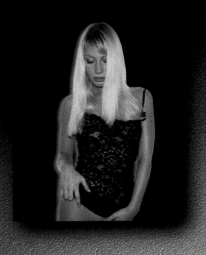

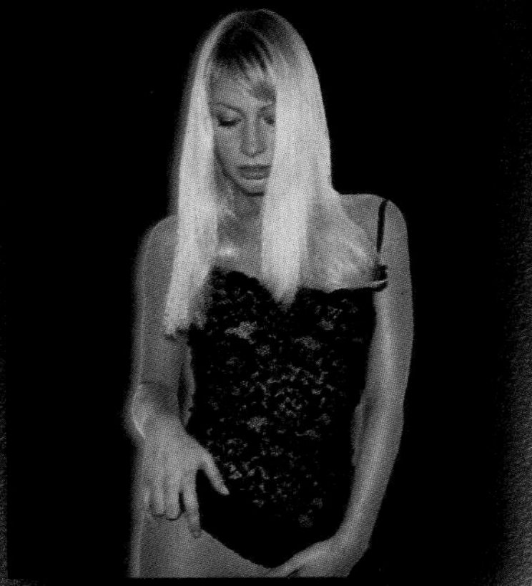

Chapter 2

SETTING THE SCENE FOR SENSUAL ENCOUNTERS

The first steps toward being adventurous in sex are developing your self-confidence and self-knowledge. The next move is to take this to your partner, in inviting them to join you in making sweet music together. But how do you set the scene for love, and how do you let your partner know what you want and what you are planning?

We often fall for the myth that says spontaneity is all. It's considered cold and calculating, unromantic and scheming to make a date to have sex. But the truth is, we actually plan ahead in our sex lives all the time, we just pretend to ourselves or our partners that sex, when it happens, is a complete surprise to us. Of course there are occasions when sex was far from your mind and you and your partner suddenly looked at each other and were overcome with desire. But be honest, how often does this happen? Most of the time, we come home knowing we're in the mood, or having even spent the whole day planning for that night's, or next morning's or even the weekend's extravaganza. Or, of course, we realize from the subtle or not so subtle hints or behaviour of our partner that they are chivvying us bedward, sooner or later. We know it's going to happen but we often dissemble, to save face. The problem is that such shyness or embarrassment can ruin a perfectly good bout of passion. If neither of you make your feelings clear, you may find the other is off the beat, not feeling up to it on that occasion. Or your partner may be thinking you aren't keen and so persuade themselves to think of something else, and be caught on the hop when you finally make your move.

THE SECRET IS IN THE PREPARATION

How do you set the scene for love, and get your partner in the mood? For some, it's a simple question of asking if they "fancy a bit". Others go the whole hog, welcoming their partner home to dimmed lights, candles, a turned-down bed and a bottle of massage oil. But letting your partner know you're in the mood for lurve, or picking up the messages they may be trying to send to you, can start earlier than this, and make lovemaking all the better for it. Indeed, setting the scene is a form of foreplay. You may have thought that foreplay was simply a delightful physical activity that was just a prelude to sex. If so, you will now have realized that the sort of non-penetrative sensual activity that we can enjoy before getting down to sexual intercourse adds a whole new dimension to sex. Foreplay doesn't merely bring you to a pitch of passion that makes sex all that more stimulating and satisfying, it is also an end in itself. The way you set yourself and your partner up for sex is similar. It enhances the eventual act, but it also is a form of satisfying love play in itself. Setting the scene is a form of flirting, and if you thought flirting was something you could do only with strangers or people with whom you're not in a relationship, think again. What flirting does is ring a bell; it signals

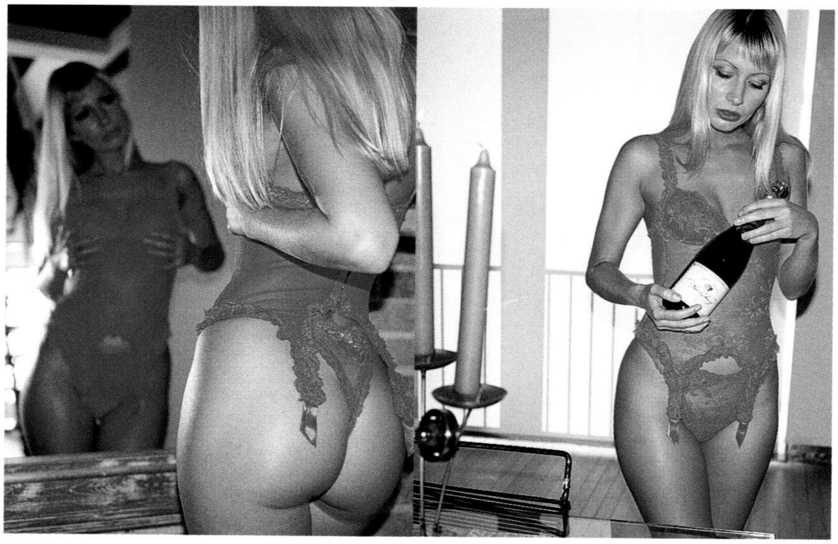

Some people go the whole hog, welcoming their partner home to dimmed lights, candles and a bottle of massage oil

Setting the scene is a form of foreplay. You may have thought that foreplay was simply a delightful physical activity that was just a prelude to sex.

interest and intent and sets an agenda. Talking of bells, this was the cue a scientist called Pavlov used when he was training dogs. He was looking at what became known as learned response. He'd ring a bell just before feeding the dogs. After a time, all he had to do was ring a bell and their mouths watered. What you and your partner may be doing is looking for ways to make sure your mouths water and you are raring to go, at a signal you'll both soon learn to recognize.

"LOOK NO HANDS!" SEX

One author has coined a phrase for what most people seem to be striving for in their sex lives. According to Erica Jong, we are all looking for the "Zipless fuck". We want it just to happen. We want our clothes to melt away without our having to struggle with zips and buttons, our contraception to be in place without our having to pause to make sure it is, the lights to dim and the bed to be turned down without our having to pause and do it. It's as if we feel that any fumbling, distraction or discussion will break the mood and ruin the whole thing. Part of setting the scene, then, is to ease you smoothly and effortlessly the whole way into each other's arms. If this is how you feel, you need to think of any element that is going to hold you up or break your concentration and so throw a wet blanket on the sex you hope to enjoy. But my view is that seeing the strings and realizing you and your partner are trying to shout "Hey, let's get it on, here!" are what make relationships close and sensual. Recognizing what you're both up to and collapsing in giggles can be the best aphrodisiac there is. What these ideas do is turn your mind lightly to thoughts of love. They don't cover up reality or make it go away.

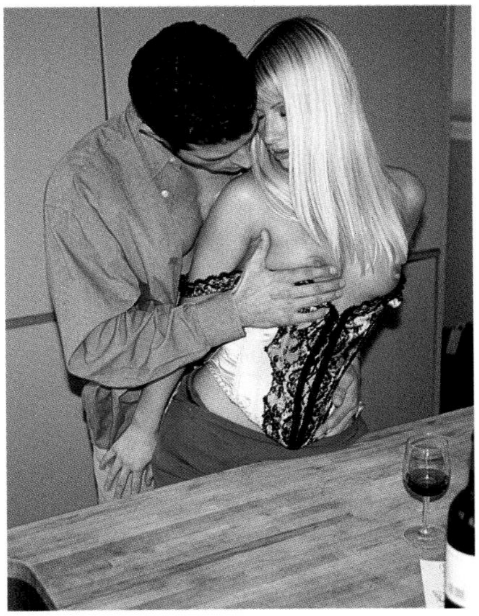

You can be raring to go when you're on the same wavelength

The key to setting the scene, preparing the way for sex, whether you do so two minutes or two days beforehand, is to be clear. Some couples like the direct approach, actually saying "I fancy making love tonight. What do you think?" Some prefer the more indirect method: "Gosh, I'd like an early night tonight. How about you?" As long as you've each deciphered the code and note what the other is talking about, euphemisms are fine. What it might mean is you and your partner learning both to send and pick up the non-verbal signals that say you're interested.

BODY LANGUAGE

Body language often sends messages that are far stronger and more effective than anything we can say. Body language is the term that describes the way our stance, gaze and hand movements reveal what is on our mind. You may not realize how much you're revealing what you're thinking, and your partner may not be able to pinpoint how it is they know. We don't always consciously recognize the messages of body language. But just as we don't realize we're saying it but still do so, we may not make out what our partner is gesturing but still get the gist of the message. But if you want to look behind the scenes and really know what is going on, here's how to tell if your partner has sex on his or her mind.

It's often not hard to see when a man is ready for sex – the average man is about as subtle with his body language as a bull in a china shop. He'll "preen" by brushing non-existent lint off his sleeves, fiddling with a tie if he's wearing one, adjusting his watch and checking his shirt cuffs. He'll turn his body toward you so, whether he's standing or sitting, his toes and knees point at you. He'll fix you with what is called the "intimate gaze", so his eyes will lock on to yours and then drift across your breasts and down your body. But if you're in any doubt, you can hardly miss the next flurry of signs. If he's really hot to trot, he'll put his thumbs in his belt so his fingers point down as if to say, "Hey, look what I've got for you." Or he'll lean back on the sofa or chair, with his legs wide apart in a wide display of his charms. Both sexes show interest by "mirroring", so if your partner is sitting or standing in exactly the same way as you – arms across the back of the sofa, legs folded under you or whatever – you know they're interested in getting in sync with you. Women show the same sort of give-away gestures, with a few extra. Women are very prone to show that toe-pointing with another twist, which is the hanging shoe. When a woman crosses her legs and sits, swinging the upper one with her shoe hanging off the toe, she may be just relaxed and comfortable. But if she's also giving out other signs it's probably a good bet she's giving her mate the come-on. Women are also likely to drop their eyes and then glance up, sideways and lick their lips, when they're in the mood. If your partner is really ready for sex, she may well show her intent by slowly crossing and uncrossing her legs while stroking her own legs. It's a hint. Take it!

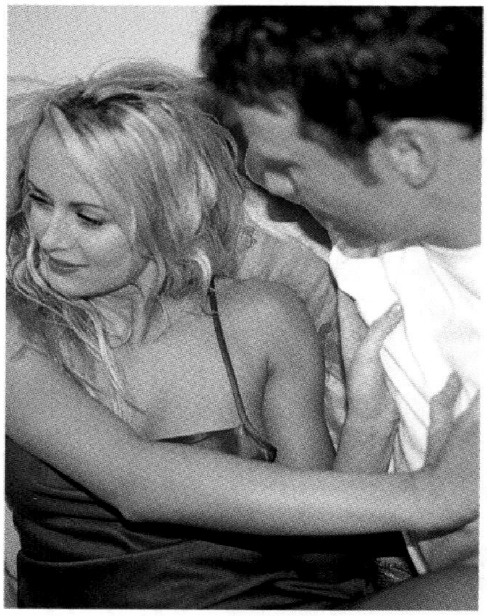

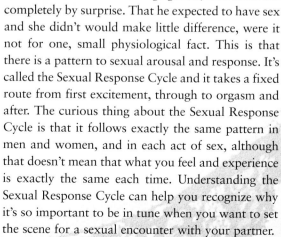

It's a real turnoff when he shows affection only when he's after sex

One important element, perhaps, is for both of you to express your sexual interest, love and affection at times other than when you want to have sex. There is nothing quite as off-putting and hurtful as the realization that the only time your partner puts an arm round you, wants a kiss or pays you any attention is when they have bed in mind. "I know when Steve wants to have sex," says Sharon. "You can hardly miss the signals because it's the only time he'll ever touch me, sometimes just about the only time he'll realize I exist. Usually, he wants his tea on the table on time, be watching telly or down the pub with his mates. When he comes home all lovey-dovey, it's because he's got sex on the brain. It really turns me off, to be honest." When a couple are used to saying, "I love you," to kissing, hugging and touching, to holding hands and talking to each other, you may need to be more specific when you want to take it further, but you won't come up against the resentful reaction of "You only do this when you want something from me!"

MAKE YOUR FEELINGS KNOWN

Making your feelings known is an important prelude because sexual desire is an elusive animal and has its own timetable. It was once believed that women were slower to arouse and less sexually interested than men. The main evidence for this was the observable fact that fewer women than men achieved sexual satisfaction from lovemaking. We'll put aside for the moment the suggestion that one reason for this could be because more men than women are poor lovers! In fact, the main reason is that, thanks to the myth that it's manly for men to be thinking about sex but unseemly for women, more men than women initiate sex. So he comes home, all hot and bothered from a hard day at work fantasizing about their evenings games, and takes her completely by surprise. That he expected to have sex and she didn't would make little difference, were it not for one, small physiological fact. This is that there is a pattern to sexual arousal and response. It's called the Sexual Response Cycle and it takes a fixed route from first excitement, through to orgasm and after. The curious thing about the Sexual Response Cycle is that it follows exactly the same pattern in men and women, and in each act of sex, although that doesn't mean that what you feel and experience is exactly the same each time. Understanding the Sexual Response Cycle can help you recognize why it's so important to be in tune when you want to set the scene for a sexual encounter with your partner.

UNDERSTANDING THE SEX CYCLE

The Sexual Response Cycle has four distinct stages. The first is arousal or excitement. This can be triggered by thinking about sex – sex with your partner, sex with a stranger, sex with a pot of chocolate mousse. It can be started by seeing or hearing something you find arousing – a sexy image, a sexy person, a sexy situation. Or it can be begun by someone touching you or making you a sexual proposition. During arousal, both men and women go through a series of physical changes. Men experience an erection, not only of the penis but sometimes of the nipples. Women too will find both their nipples and their clitoris are likely to swell, as does the labia or area round the vagina. They'll also experience some moisture in the vagina as a prelude to sex.

Arousal is a real piece of string; it can last as long as you want, or can sometimes be a stage you gallop through in minutes. It is followed by the second phase, the Plateau stage. Plateau is a bit like the moment on a roller coaster where you reach the top of the first big drop. It's the point during which you catch a breath because you know, any moment now, you're going to need it. During Plateau, both men and women will flush, not just on their faces but also on chest, stomach, shoulders and arms. It's why women put on blusher to appear attractive and why that "just out of the gym or off the track" sweaty look is such a turn on. There is nothing quite as attractive as someone who looks as if they're hot and bothered at the sight of you. Both men and women will find the sexual parts of their bodies will increase in size – not just nipples and penis, but also breasts and balls. Blood pressure will have increased, your pulse will be racing and you'll be breathing fast. Once you reach plateau you know, barring a halt in the proceedings, that the third stage, Orgasm, is only thirty seconds to three minutes away. When the point of orgasmic inevitability is reached, it happens and you can't stop it. During Orgasm, you'll be panting and your heart will be pounding. Your body will also be overtaken with a series of muscular contractions that you won't be able to control. Following Orgasm is the fourth stage, Resolution, during which all the changes that have happened return to normal in reverse order. The flush that has spread across your body recedes, the swollen and enlarged areas of your body decrease again and your breathing and heart rate go back to normal.

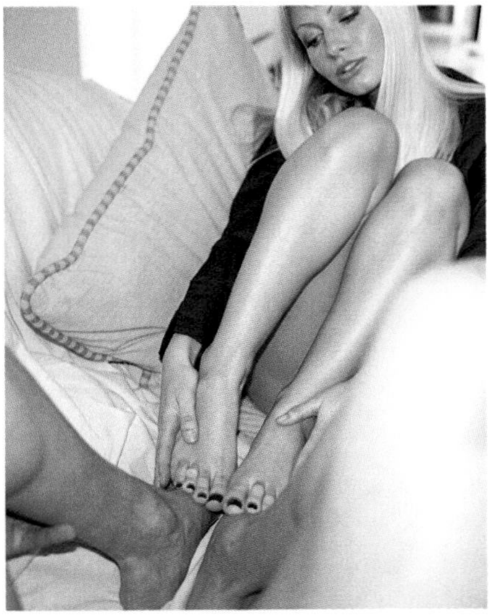

Being in touch with each other makes love better

STEALING A MARCH

The cycle is the same in men and women, and the same each time you make love. What you actually feel and how far along the cycle you proceed, and how quickly, may, however, alter each time. Arousal, as mentioned, can last anything from several hours to a few minutes. You can interrupt or hold yourself back at Plateau and so never reach orgasm. And some people, having experienced orgasm, go on to another plateau and further orgasms before reaching resolution. But the important element to concentrate on here is the role of arousal. If one of you is already excited by the time you and your partner start making love, or is someone who can and does move swiftly on through this stage, this time or every time, you may leave your partner trailing well behind you. And if you jump immediately into having penetrative sex and roll over and go to sleep afterward, it's hardly surprising your partner may be left staring at the ceiling, wondering if that's all there is to it. It's not that one of you is slow or frigid, it's because one of you stole a march and never let the other catch up. So, that's why it's so important to let each other know what you're thinking, what you're wanting and how, when and where you'd like to get it on. The aim is either to

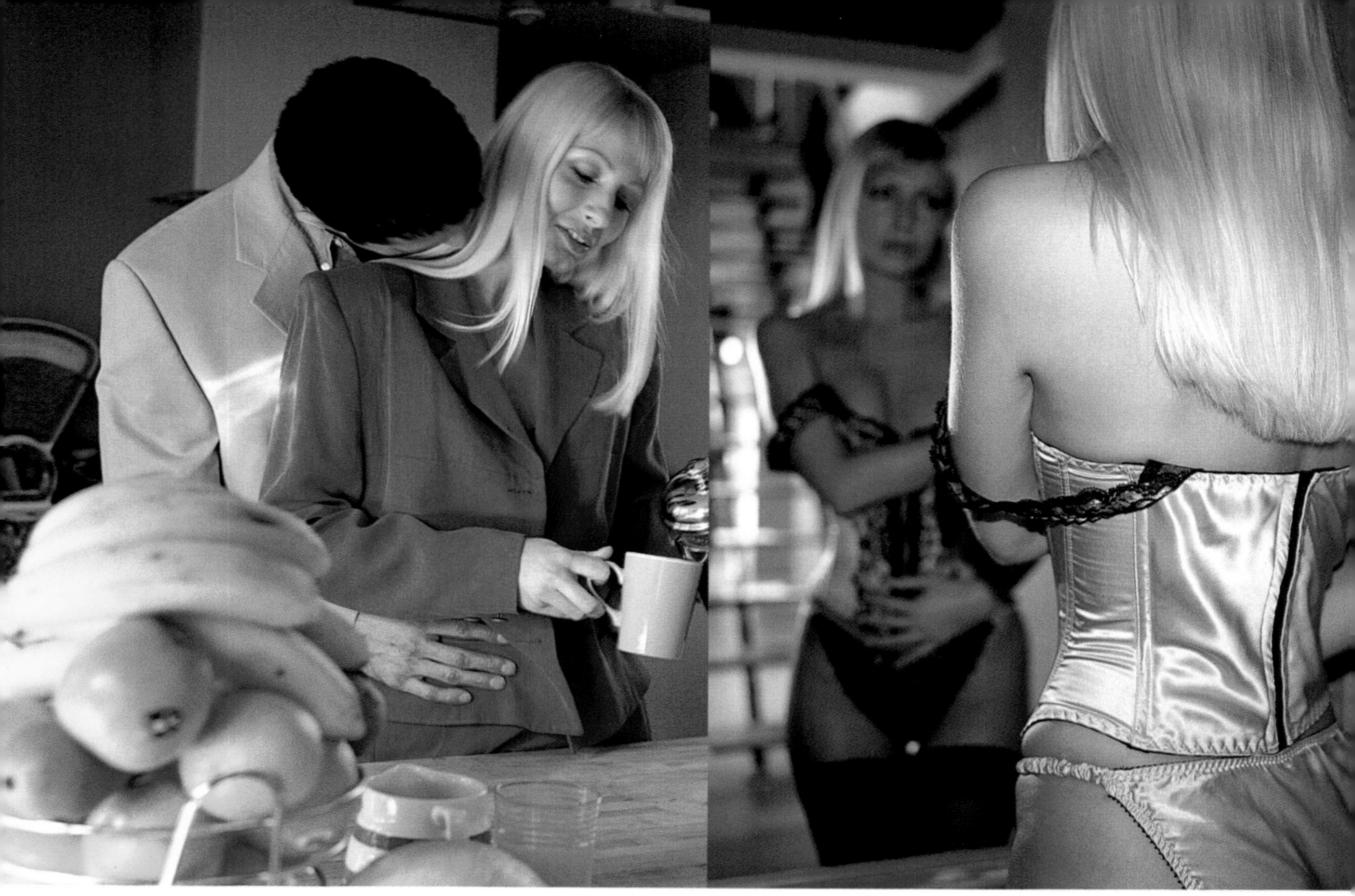

A kiss over breakfast can lead to lovemaking that night

match your patterns so that both of you are at roughly the same stage of arousal, can be at Plateau and then on to Orgasm together. Or that one of you can linger in the arousal stage, which you can prolong for a considerable time, until the other catches up. Or one of you, having gone through Plateau to Orgasm, can then concentrate on your partner until they too reach their end point. And, let's face it, even when both of you have had an orgasm, that doesn't have to be the end point at all. It's not just that both of you may find a capacity for more than one orgasm, there is also the fact that many people enjoy slow and gentle caresses even more after they've had a fast and furious orgasm.

I have said that the cycle is the same in men and women and the same each time you make love. By that I mean that, all things being equal, both of you will go from arousal through plateau to orgasm and resolution. However, the cycle can be interrupted, leaving either of you high, dry and frustrated. If you become aroused and don't have an orgasm it takes far longer than the two or three minutes of resolution for the flushed and swollen parts of your body to return to normal. You'll feel sore and aching – a phenomenon boys call "blue balls". And if lovemaking has been particularly prolonged, exciting and adventurous, your experience of the pleasures of orgasm, and indeed of the whole experience, will be that much greater. To paraphrase Orwell, "All orgasms are equal but some are more equal than others".

GETTING IT TOGETHER

So you can see how important it is to let your partner know – and to be honest with yourself – about your sexual desires. On one level it's to ensure that you get some satisfaction. But going a whole lot higher, the more prepared you are, the more both of you are going to enjoy it. So let's look at this idea of spontaneity in sex. Why should we be shy and embarrassed at finding a partner attractive and anticipating having sex with them? It may be fine to decide at the drop of a hat to have quick and sudden sex which could be all the more exciting for catching you unawares. That's a bit like deciding to go down to the local store for a take-away. But a total diet of wham-bam-thank-you- Sam sex, like a total diet of convenience food, ain't good for the waistline or the relationship. So you've got to look upon some of your sex life as being the special meal, the celebratory dinner for two or even the over-the-top banquet, and to draw up your shopping list and plan for it in exactly the same way. We often keep quiet and hold ourselves back when we do have an impulse to show affection to a partner. We feel like kissing the back of their neck, stroking an arm or hugging them and we feel foolish and do nothing. Or we would like to say "I love you" or maybe even "I really fancy you tonight", and then other people and other demands get in the way. So the first rule is to go with your feelings. The next time you feel like it, just do it. One reason we may hold back, of course, is the possible reactions of our partners. We fear rejection, so when they pull away or tell you not to be so soft, we can feel hurt and unwelcome. But it's often their own embarrassment that makes them act this way, not any reflection on you. So don't take it personally, but persist.

How can you start sending out the signals that say you are sexually interested to your partner? And how indeed do you pick up on the signals they may be sending you? And, how early can you start? There is a whole range of ways of doing this, from the glaringly obvious to the whisperingly discreet. Next time you have made love close your eyes and think back to what made you realize, or how your partner may have realized, that sex was in the offing. Was it because you took particular care about the clothes you were wearing or the cologne you put on? Was it because you made a particular fuss about them or changed your routine that morning, that evening or that day? Whether you realized it or not, there would have been something in your behaviour that signalled sex was in mind long before either of you made the offer. If so, make a point of doing that again and see how the other responds. But the obvious move can often bring the greatest rewards. Make up your mind that you and your partner are going to make love at a particular point this evening, tomorrow or on the weekend and start planning for the event. You can plan for love two hours, two days or even two weeks in advance – the longer the advance warning, the greater the opportunity you have to get prepared.

> *To be in the mood to accept an invitation for sex, it's a good idea to lay the foundation way back before sex is even on your mind.*

START EARLY

If you want your partner to be in the mood to accept an invitation for sex, it's a good idea to lay the foundation way back before sex is even on your mind. To do this, try to make a habit of letting your partner know how much you love them. A kiss here, a kiss there, a stroke, a hug and a caress all get the point across. Find things about which you can compliment them, to make them feel good about themselves, whether it's their appearance or something they may have done. If the groundwork has been done in advance, it's that much easier to get what you want, when you want it. Come the right time, plan your campaign and start to carry it out.

There are times when surprising your partner and catching them unawares may make for good loving. But unless both of you have established a framework for picking up on each other's desires, this could lead to disappointment. There's nothing quite as hurtful as having slaved away all day to welcome your lover into your bed and your arms and to have them look at a candle-lit dinner for two and demand "What's up? Someone special coming for dinner? And is there a power cut again?" This is one reason why it's a good idea to make it very clear what you would like to happen.

To prepare the ground, you could slip a note into your partner's pocket or place it in or on any form of diary they carry, paper or electronic. It could be a love poem or simply a suggestion for what you would like to do to or with them – romantic or downright obscene! Or you might put something a bit more specific where they will find it somewhere in the day, such as a condom, a bottle of massage oil, a feather or a pair of handcuffs with an attached suggestion that they might like to use it with you later. If you are not going to be together and your partner is someone who would be horribly embarrassed if a friend or colleague saw any of this, be discreet. But actually most people would be only too pleased to be shown up as being highly desirable red-hot lovers who inspire so much lust in their partner's eyes. You may get the best result if you arrange for your love letter to fall out in front of other people during a coffee break.

It's a bit of a cliché to suggest that a wife should be waiting at the door in a negligee with a martini in her hand, not to say sexist. But I have to say that it works.

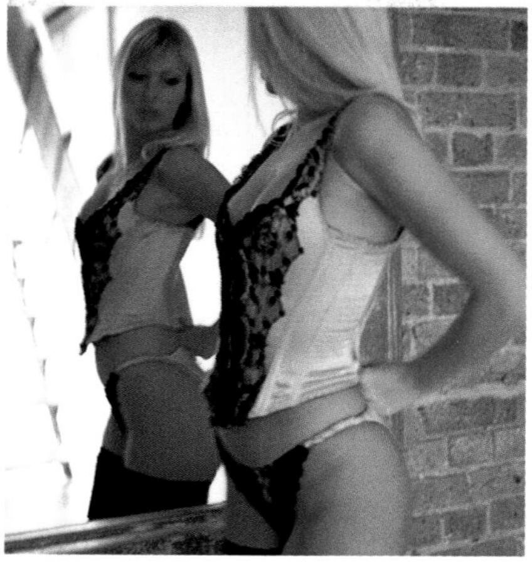

Welcome your partner home

I JUST CALLED TO SAY …

If you are apart during the day, make a point of getting in contact by phone or by e-mail. Make the first contact non-specific. Say something along the lines of "I just thought I'd let you know I love you and am missing you and am looking forward to seeing you tonight." Call a second time later and this time introduce the subject of sex. You could say, "I was just thinking about the last time we made love and I can't wait for the next time." With the third call set up your rendezvous and make a date for whenever it is you would like to get down and dirty.

You can seduce your partner in the bedroom or living room, in ordinary clothes and after a cup of tea, as a sort of afterthought when you reach the correct moment. But if you really want to prolong the foreplay and pump up the volume, put some effort into announcing your intentions and making the surroundings and atmosphere fit what is on your mind. It's a bit of a cliché to suggest that a wife should be waiting at the door in a negligee with a martini in her hand, not to say sexist. But I have to say that it works – even more if he's the one to be waiting by the door, in his cycling shorts with a glass of chilled Chardonnay at the ready! Paying attention to what your partner finds when they come home, or when you come home to them, can make the difference between a loving encounter and a total anticlimax. If you've problems or issues that need to be raised or discussed, either put them away until another time or deal with them together well before you want to start the lovemaking. If it's sex you want and sex you will have, make sure that sex and romance are the only things on your mind and on the agenda, and in the conversation.

To prepare the ground, you could slip a note into your partner's pocket or place it in or on any form of diary they carry, paper or electronic. If you are apart during the day, make a point of getting in contact by phone or by e-mail.

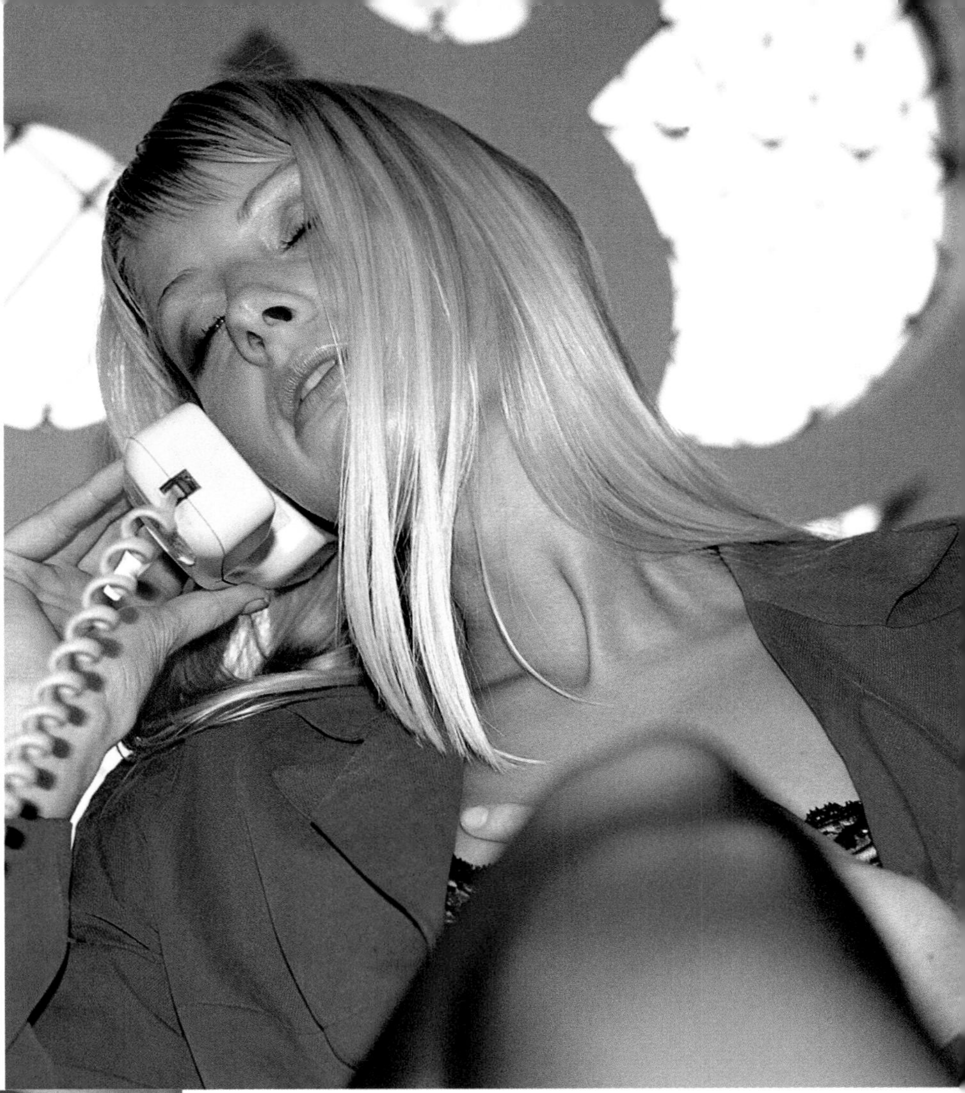

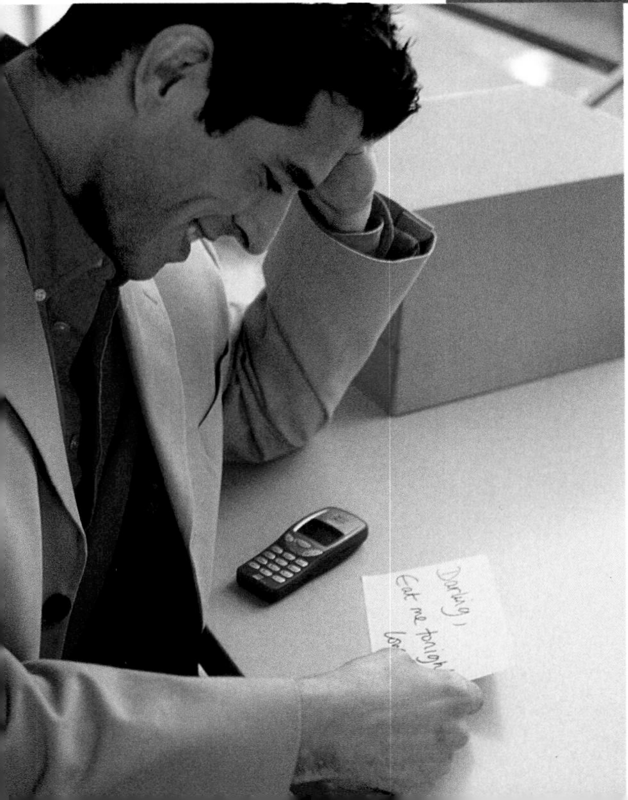

A phone call or a note can tell your partner to expect fireworks later on!

SUPER-SENSITIVITY

Set up your room to suggest that sensual adventures are in the offing. Sexual arousal has the effect of making you super-sensitive to physical sensations. Appealing to all your senses is one way of getting yourselves in the mood. Turn the heating up or run a hot bath into which you'll invite your partner. You really can't be expected to shed your clothes if it's freezing cold. Dim the lights, or throw a scarf over table lights and drape them over ceiling lights, or simply place candles everywhere. There is a good reason why dim and flickering light gives a sexual boost. This is because quite literally the first sign of sexual arousal in either gender is the dilation or widening of the pupil. Pupils also widen when it's darker. If you look at someone in bright light, when their pupils are contracted, they don't seem terribly interested in you. Look at them in candle light and all of a sudden it appears that they have got the absolute hots for you, which is the biggest come-on of all time.

Many couples find that incense is a particularly potent way of starting off, with its aura of exotic mystery and Eastern delights. If you don't like incense, try a spray of your favourite perfume or cologne or have a bowl of potpourri and stir it up when you want the smell to fill the room. Mood music can also do the trick, or sounds that you find particularly evocative – the sound of waves on the shore, waterfalls, bird song or the grand prix if that's what jerks your strings! Touch is a particularly important sense and you may like to offer your partner a massage to relax them. You can do this as a prelude to sex or as foreplay. Alternatively, massage each other well before, and separate from, love making. The pleasures of touch, of the laying on of hands that takes place during a massage, can be a pleasure in itself. It's a way of reacquainting yourself with your partner's body, of giving and receiving pleasure just for its own sake. It can be a delicious way of heralding sex but it can sometimes be even better to use it to relax and energise each other several hours before you move from the sensual to the sexual.

To give a really exotic and erotic massage, make your partner comfortable by spreading out a washable sheet or towel on the floor or bed and inviting them to lie back and put themselves in your hands. Make sure your hands are warm – you could dunk them in hot water to chase away any surface chill.

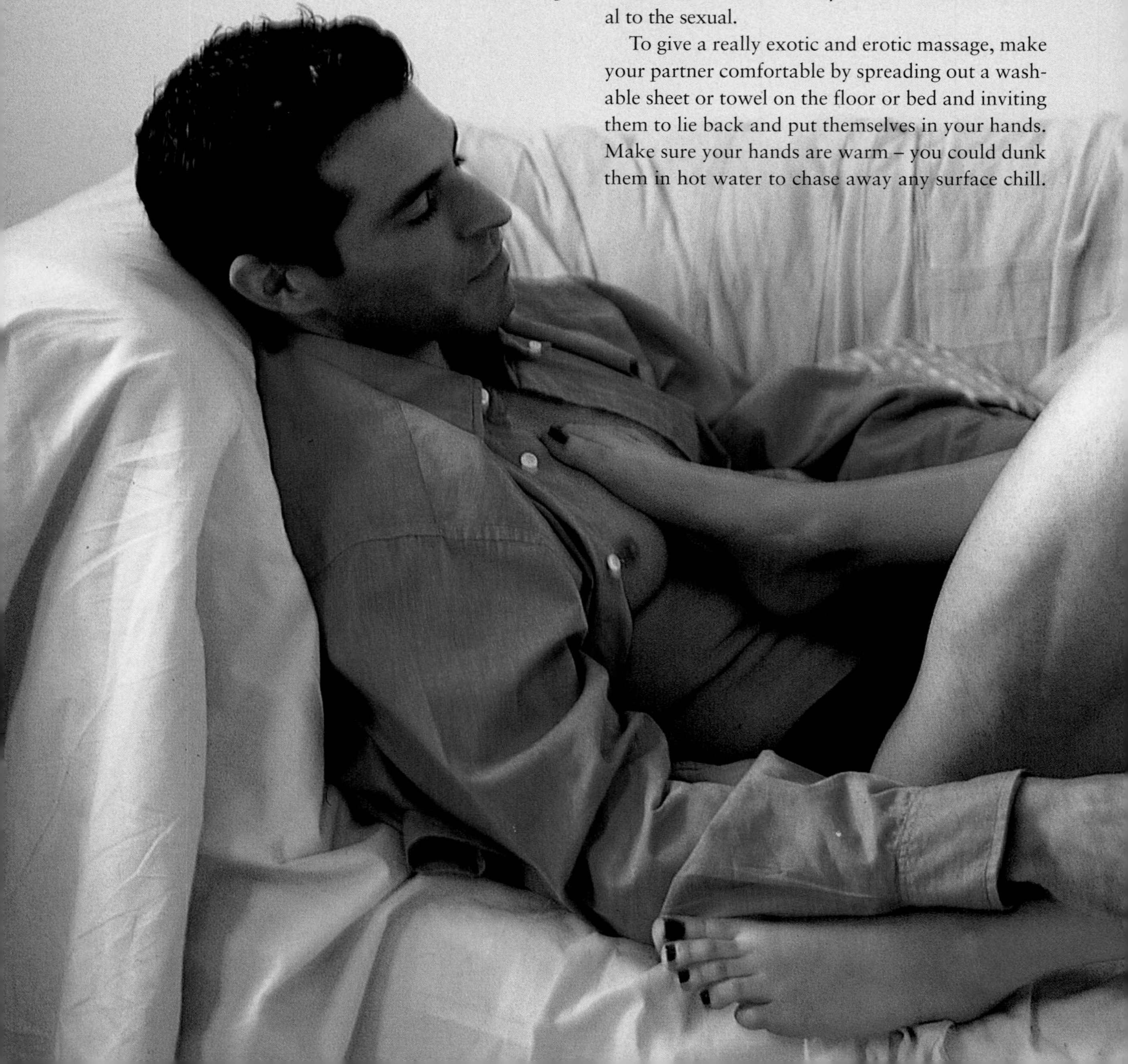

Pour a generous handful of cream or oil into your palms and rub them together to warm up the lotion before beginning. Ask your partner to lie on their stomach and sit astride them, being careful about how much weight you bear down. Begin with your partner's back, stroking and rubbing the neck and shoulders. In turn, rub gently down each arm, brushing the inside of the elbows and manipulating and stroking hands and fingers. Return to the back and knead round the shoulder blades and down the backbone, down to the small of their back. Sweep your hands over and around the buttocks before descending down the legs to the toes. Pay especial attention to the inside of the thighs and the backs of the knees. When you've reached the soles of their feet, ask them to turn over and go back up their body, from feet to chest. Rub, stroke and knead, listening to your partner's responses to get directions from them as to what feels good. When you've tired yourself out and they feel as loose and relaxed as a cat in front of a log fire, rest your hands on them for a moment and take a breather. Then, it's your turn to be pampered. Change places and have them do the same to you. If just touching each other has you excited and raring to go and you can't wait till later for sex, when you gently pass up from the feet, you will bring

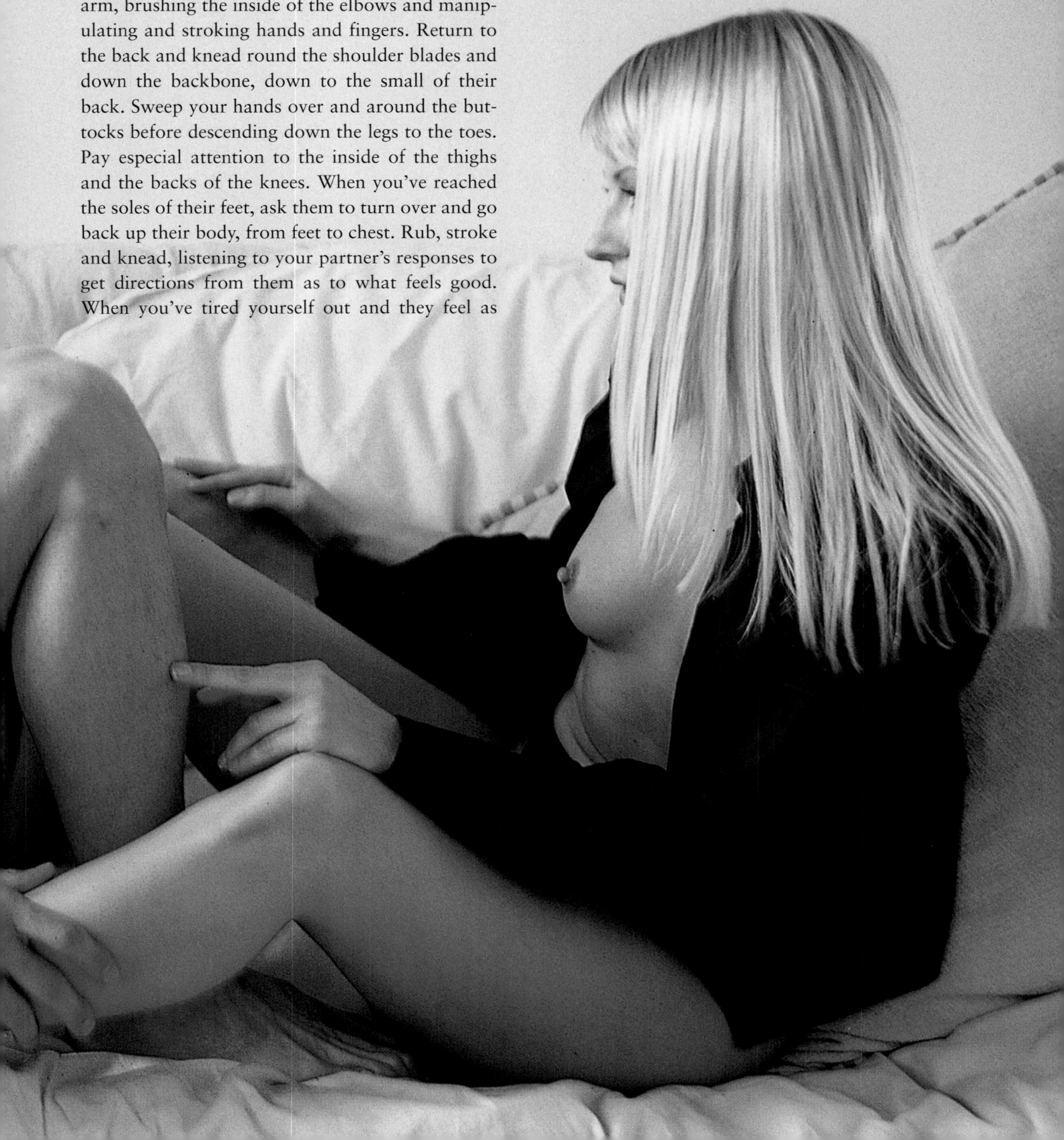

sexual caresses into play. Make sure your hands are covered in oil or cream as you gently and then more firmly stroke your partner's body and genitals. The masseuse/masseur can ask that the other either gives them a soothing and reviving body rub after you've made love, or that they can be the one to lie back next time.

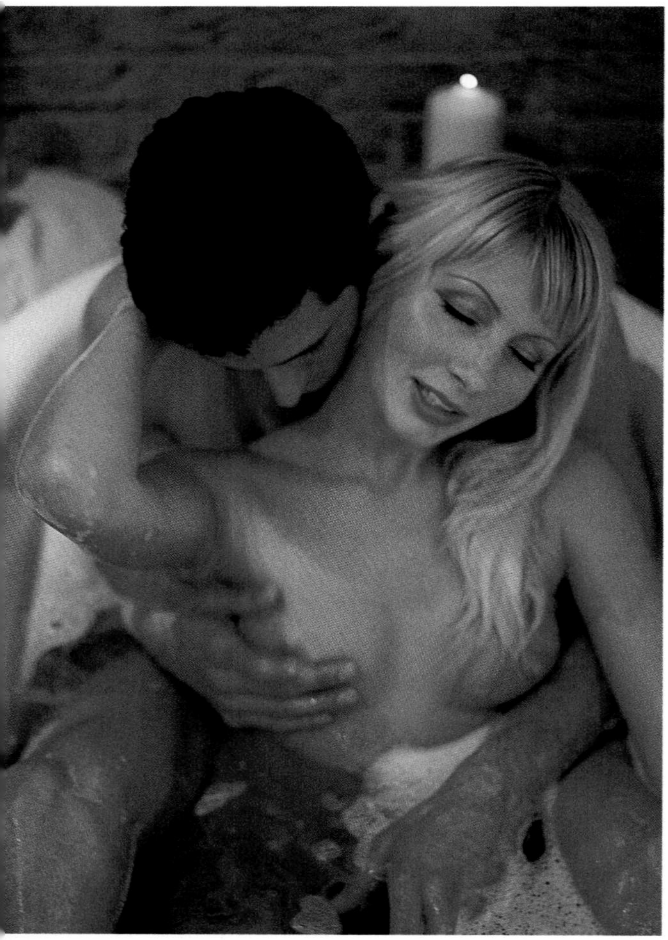

Pamper your partner with an erotic massage

WASH YOUR BLUES AWAY

You could also offer your partner a sensual bath to put both of you in the mood. Line every safe and available surface with candles and turn the lights out. Make your bath hot, full and outrageously scented with oils or bath gel. You could also use herbal mixtures. Basil, bayleaf, lavender, lemon verbena, lovage, meadowsweet, rosemary, sage and thyme are supposed to be particularly stimulating. Catnip, camomile, jasmine, limeflower and vervaine are supposed to be relaxing. Most of these come in sachets or as tea bags. Just throw a few of your chosen ones into your bath. Black pepper, cardamom, jasmine, juniper, orange blossom, patchouli, clary sage, rose, sandalwood or ylang-ylang are supposed to be particularly sexy, and come as essential oils. You can burn them as incense or use the oil sparingly in a burner or in the bath itself. Use a brush or a loofah and plenty of shower gel or soap to work up a lather and get your skin tingling. Follow up with soft flannels and sponges to soothe and smooth. While you are teasing and satisfying all your other senses, think about your taste buds too. Tantalize your partner with thoughts of using their lips on you by first feeding them tiny and luscious tit-bits, the more luxurious the better. Asparagus spears, quail eggs, smoked salmon, slices of fresh fig and melon will all put you in the mood by having you think of parts of the body that look or feel similar. An exotic, sensual feast in an Arabian Nights scenario is a popular fantasy for many people. In chapter 7, we'll be making specific suggestions for how you can use that to brighten up your lovelife. Finish off by wrapping each other in large, warm towels before inviting your partner to step through into the bedroom to take advantage of your by now thoroughly warmed and relaxed state. Of course, if you can't wait you could throw a towel on the

Line every safe and available surface with candles and turn the lights out. Make your bath hot, full and outrageously scented with oils or bath gel.

bathroom floor or even try sex standing up. The truly athletic and supple may even have sex in the bath. Just have a thought for Health and Safety Regulations and be careful you neither slip nor drown!

LET ME TAKE YOU AWAY FROM ALL THIS

But if you want to make a very definite statement to your partner that sex is top of your plans for this weekend or evening, there are two ways you can let them know, with no room for confusion or doubt. One is to spirit them away from your boring, humdrum existence for just a little while. It's often easy to get out of the habit of having a wild, passionate love life while you're at home. You sleep together, rather than having sex together, more nights than not, and when you come home it's often to routine and chores that have to be done. So, if you can afford the money or the time, taking your partner away for a night is an ideal way of putting sex very firmly on the agenda. Knowing you are going to be in a hotel room with a ready-made double bed (and do make sure you ask for a double, not twins) that you are not going to have to tidy up yourself the following morning can really get the juices flowing. Hotel rooms are frequently ideal for sexy assignations – all those free lotions and potions in the en-suite bathroom with constant hot water – in a room that always seems dominated by The Bed, in anonymity and privacy. You are on your own, you are not going to be interrupted or overheard and even if you are you can just walk out and leave it behind you the next day. But most important of all, both of you know that a night or a weekend away is dedicated to sex and you can enjoy working yourselves and each other up to it from the moment you book until the moment you get there.

PILLOW BOOKS

Another way of making your wishes, ideas and plans clear to your partner is to use some very upfront visual clues to give them a bit more than a hint. Most of us can be interested and indeed aroused by the thought, sound or sight of other people's bodies and of other people's lovemaking. This is why "pillow books" and erotic texts have always been popular from the time cave-dwellers drew pictures on their cave walls to show each other how to do it. The erotic arts now come in the form of videos and Internet sites as well as films, books and magazines. We often turn to erotica to give us or our partners a hint or a reminder, to let them know we're keen to have sex or to get ourselves going. We may want specific ideas for sexual positions or sexual variations or we may want something to stimulate our private fantasies, whether for our eyes only or to share with our partners. Some erotic material is made specifically for the purpose of arousing us, but let's be truthful here, high art and culture can have just as much of a stimulating effect.

There continues to be a debate over whether pornographic material degrades and corrupts and

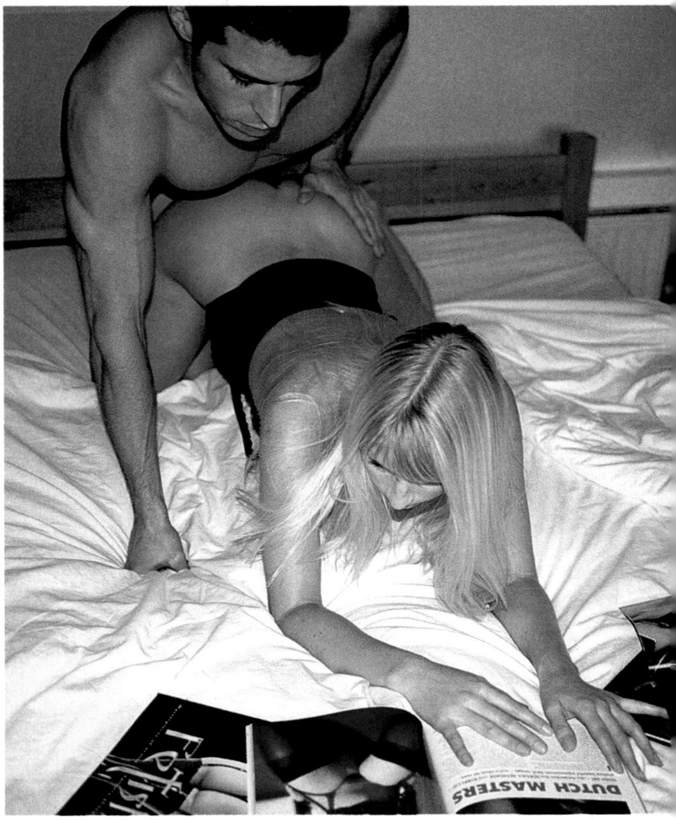

Other people's bodies can put you in the mood

leads to abusive behaviour. But sexually explicit material is seen by millions of people every day who have not, do not and never would be abusive. Surely the impact of erotica has to do with what

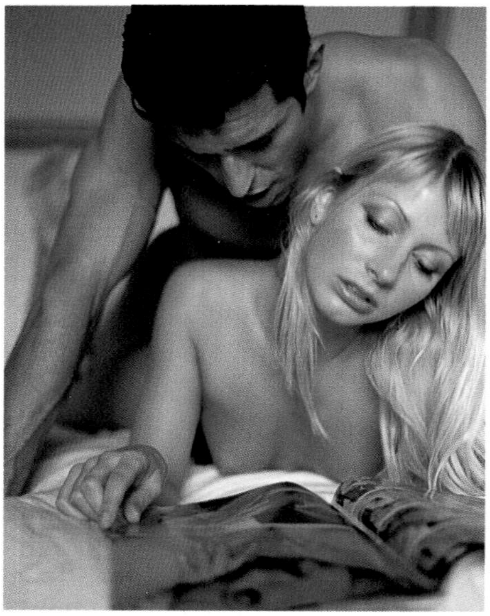

"Pillow books" are a centuries-old tradition

satisfaction. There are currently plenty of films on general release as well as specifically made blue movies that couples can find to be a lift to their sex lives. You could plan a video night to see what you and your partner might find appealing. Make sure you will be alone and undisturbed and each of you pick a video you would like. You could, of course, go for a purpose-made pornographic movie but you are just as likely to find there are plenty of standard films that have scenes that are exciting to you. Wear sexy clothes, dim the lights and start the film. Snuggle close and when a scene that excites you comes on let your partner know how you feel about it. You can rewind to pick out extra pointers and use the action on the screen as a mirror for yourselves.

PUT YOURSELF IN THE PICTURE

If sight and sound seems to be the route for you, you can go a step further by doing things for yourself

There are currently plenty of films on general release as well as specifically made blue movies that couples can find to be a lift to their sex lives.

exactly it shows and how and why you use it? If what you are seeing is consensual sex in the context of equality and respect for others, then it is acceptable. Recent studies confirm that women can be just as aroused as men by explicit material. It used to be thought that women preferred romantic written material and weren't particularly aroused by the more explicit or the visual. In fact, the difference is explained more by the material available than by the difference in the responses of the sexes. The point is that, until recently, most erotica was by men for men or by men for their fantasy of what women would like. It's not surprising that most women, and quite a few men, find this a turn off. Women are often presented not as people with their own sexual desires and with whom men share lovemaking, but as objects with which a man can achieve his own excitement and

Right: For private viewing only

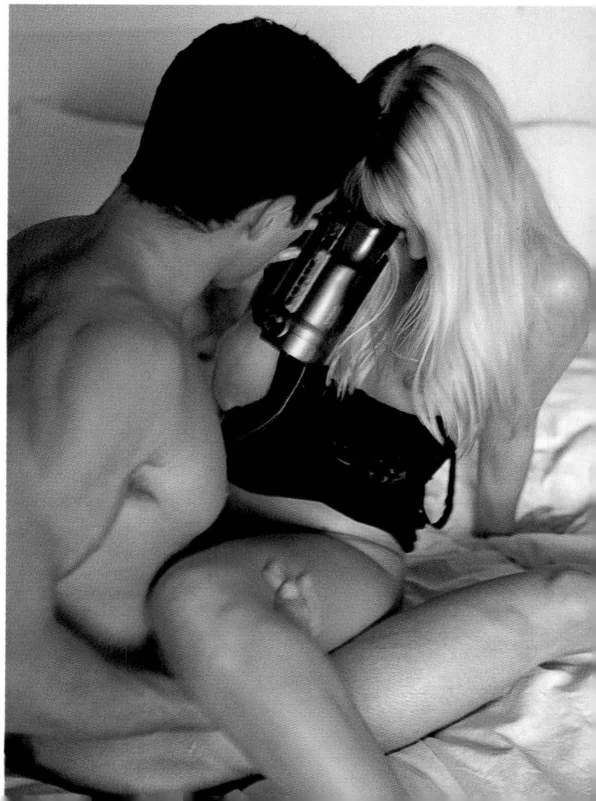

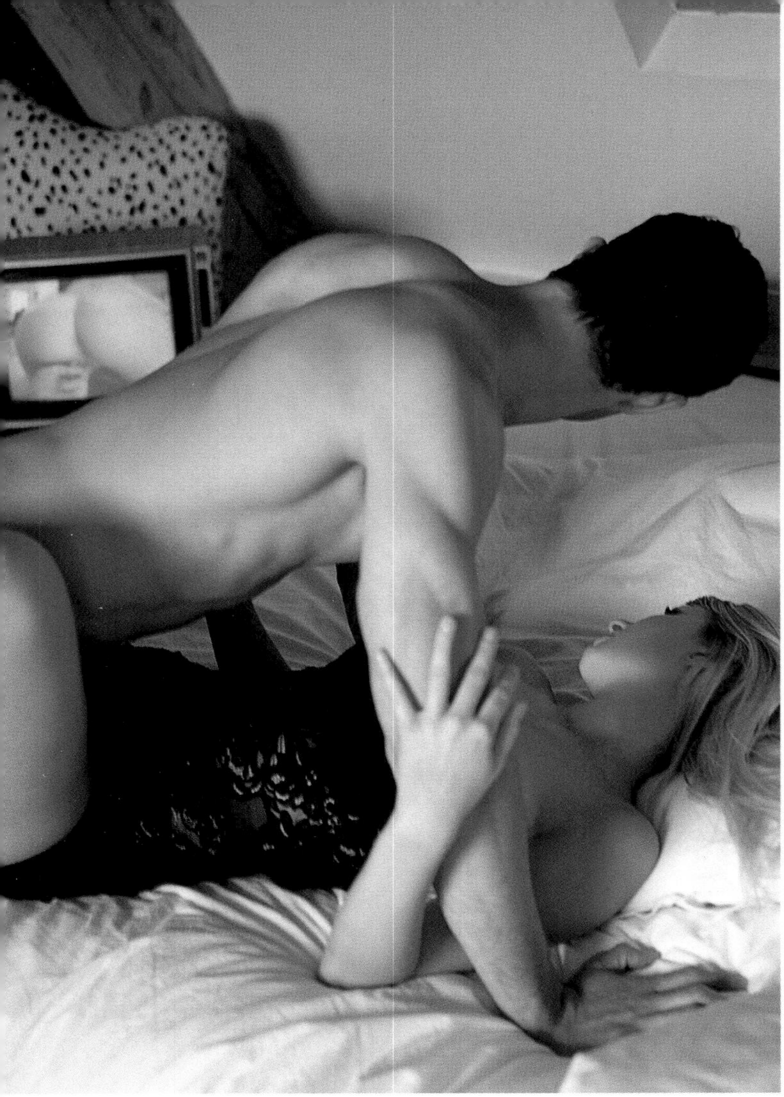

Sights and sounds add to your own pleasure

and making photographs, tapes or videos of yourself and your partner in action. Many people find the thought of being on camera and in front of an audience a turn-on. Others feel the sight or the sound of themselves and their partner having sex to be highly arousing. You might then find re-runs of a past experience are all you need both to set you off and heighten your next one. You could use a Polaroid camera or camcorder or a tape recorder to capture the sight or sound of your lovemaking. Next time you are feeling like making love, bring the equipment out and it's more than likely to put your partner in the mood too. You could also use mirrors to give you a view of yourselves while in action. Dim the lights in your bedroom, perhaps just leaving a door ajar to give some faint illumination from a hallway light or having a few candles to give a flickering light. Angle a floor-length mirror to catch your own image on the bed, or prop open the wardrobe door if that's where you keep your mirror. If you find this does the trick, you could tile an entire wall or even your ceiling above the bed to give you a new viewpoint on love.

Polaroid or video or sound tapes, which you make yourself, are perfectly legal as long as they are strictly for your own use. But be careful and do keep them to yourselves. If you send them through the post, you could be charged with sending indecent material by mail. If you take photographs on ordinary film and have them developed for you, you could also fall foul of the law. Most developing and printing is done automatically and so they may be unseen by human eye, but if anyone does see them they can report you to the police and, if nothing else, it could be highly embarrassing for you.

You don't expect a party or any sort of special occasion to go with a swing without forward planning and preparation. Successful loving is no different, even if it does happen a bit more often than a Millennium party. Just because you make love several times a year, you shouldn't get complacent. If you treated each time as a special occasion, arranging the scene as carefully as you would lay your table and set out decorations for a celebration meal, you would find it pays. Set the scene for sex, and you'll find sex sets you up for maximum pleasure.

Polaroid or video or sound tapes, which you make yourself, are perfectly legal as long as they are strictly for your own use.

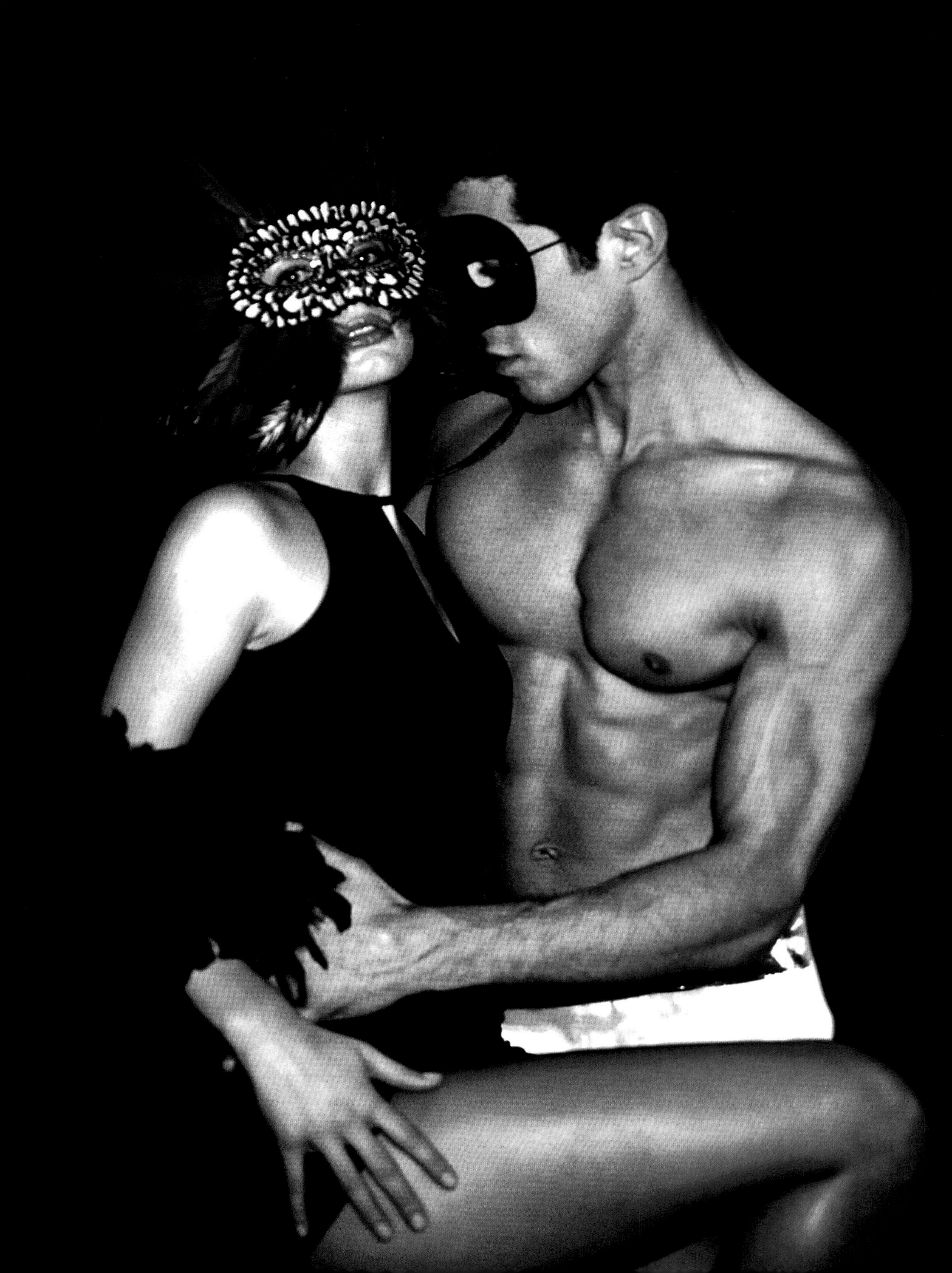

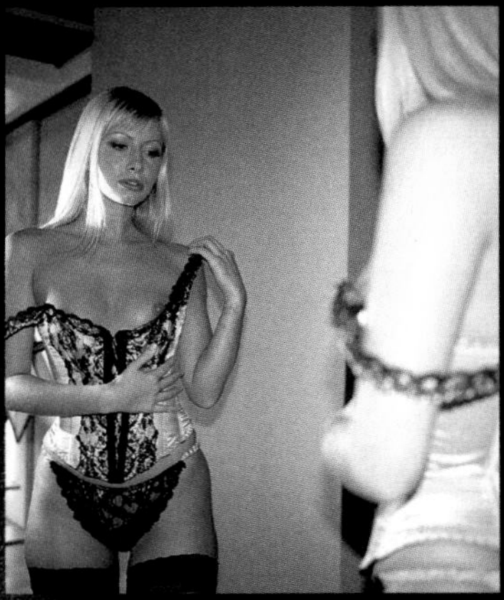

Chapter 3

DRESSING FOR SEX

To feel sexy you need to feel confident about yourself, and for most of us an important component of self-confidence is feeling good about our appearance. Sadly, many people go down the dead end of thinking they have to look conventionally pretty or handsome to be appealing. The truth is that if you fall in love with someone and they with you it's your own individual looks that appeal.

She may think that she's a few pounds overweight, he may fear he's a tad lacking in the hair department, but the reason you are together is because he likes something to get hold of and she has a thing about slap heads. If you feel you don't match up to what you think of as the ideal man or woman, don't despair. Few real people do, and the models we admire and envy and try to copy are not in themselves all that they might seem. The bodies you see in the papers and magazines, either in advertisements or modelling clothes, often look the way they do because of lots of artificial help. Transparent tape is used to hold breasts in gravity-defying uplifts. Those wonderful full and erect nipples that are the despair of the "normal" woman stand up like that because of ice cubes, a cold water spray or a quick tweak with the fingers as the shutter clicks. If you've never understood why yours are flat or even dimpled except when you're sexually aroused, while theirs seem to stand out all the time, now you know how they do it. Make-up, air-brushing and other digital or direct tinkering with the negatives gets rid of veins, stretch marks and other blemishes. Men tend to look so very manly because he either puts a sock in it or gives himself a quick feel. With a side view from the camera and skilful lighting, a tiny sausage can become a mighty salami in the picture! In real life, away from the photographer's tricks, most male models are no different from the rest.

Rather than trying to change the essential you, the art is to present yourself in the best possible light and that means dressing to kill and thrill. There's another aspect to dressing up for sexy adventures. This is that we all have sexual fantasies – dreams and scenarios that enliven our imaginations when it comes to thinking about sex. You can use your clothing and the accessories that go with it to bring these to life. All it needs is the self-confidence to start.

DRESS TO THRILL

Begin by looking through your own wardrobe and having a think about what you've got that actually puts you in the mood. What clothing do you already possess that, when you put it on, makes you feel "tonight's the night"? It could be something that you associate with a memorably sexual encounter when your partner really came on strong to you. The chances are that this is something your partner finds especially arousing or it could be something that gives you a boost. When you put it on you feel there is no saying no to you tonight, and this makes you strut your stuff, sending a "come on" to your partner.

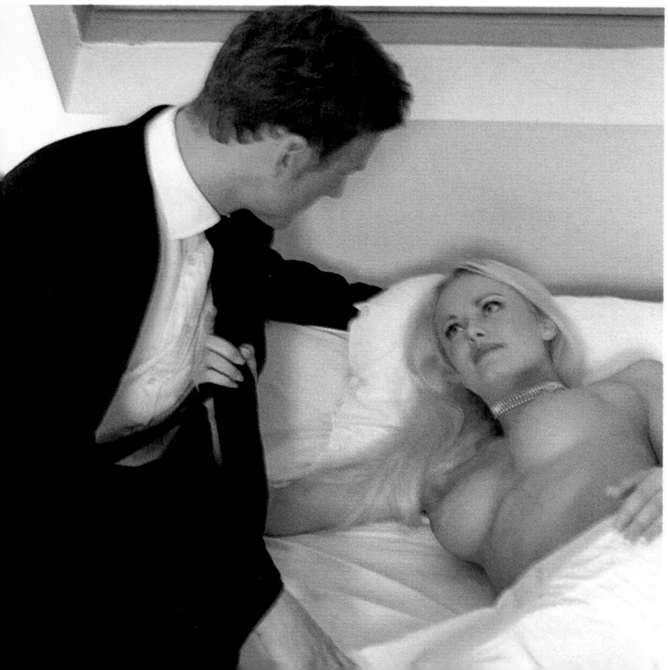

Some articles of clothing are fairly obviously sexual in nature. Plunging necklines, leather, velvet and anything tight and clingy are likely to do it for both sexes. High heels on women and large belt buckles on men often send an exceptionally sexual signal. The trick is finding what in particular tickles your own fancy and that of your partner. You may find, for instance, that articles that may not at first seem arousing have a particular effect on one or other of you. One person, for instance, may find a fleecy jacket has a special resonance. Another that chokers or bow ties say "come and get me". Look at your own wardrobe but then explore with your partner what they like you wearing and what you may like to shop for.

Common favourites are anything with fur or fleece, leather, silk, velvet and satin, or their look-alikes, which can all have you panting for a touch. What they all share is texture. Thinking back to our earliest days and our earliest memories, not just our own but our ancestral remembrances, it's the natural textures of skin and fur that make us feel comforted and secure. Slide your hands over slinky satin or warm and silky velvet and you are likely to find the hairs on the back of your neck standing to attention – as well as other parts of your body! You can harness this natural response by making sure something in your outfit just calls to your partner to come and stroke.

Clothing also sends certain messages by summoning up a time or a place. If you and your partner have a specific memory of a passionate interlude on holiday, walking into the bedroom wearing a shirt or blouse or swimming costume that you wore then will bring not only the memories but the sexual arousal flooding back. Or you can recall the special intensity of your early days together by digging out an article you might have worn on your first date, or the first time you "did it" together. You can also find clothes that say something particular about your sexual interests. Put on a baby-doll nightdress or a pair of soccer shorts if either of you has a hankering to be seduced as a fresh young innocent by an older partner, and you could be pleasantly surprised at the reaction.

Left: Some people may find that the wearing of chokers or bow ties says "come and get me"

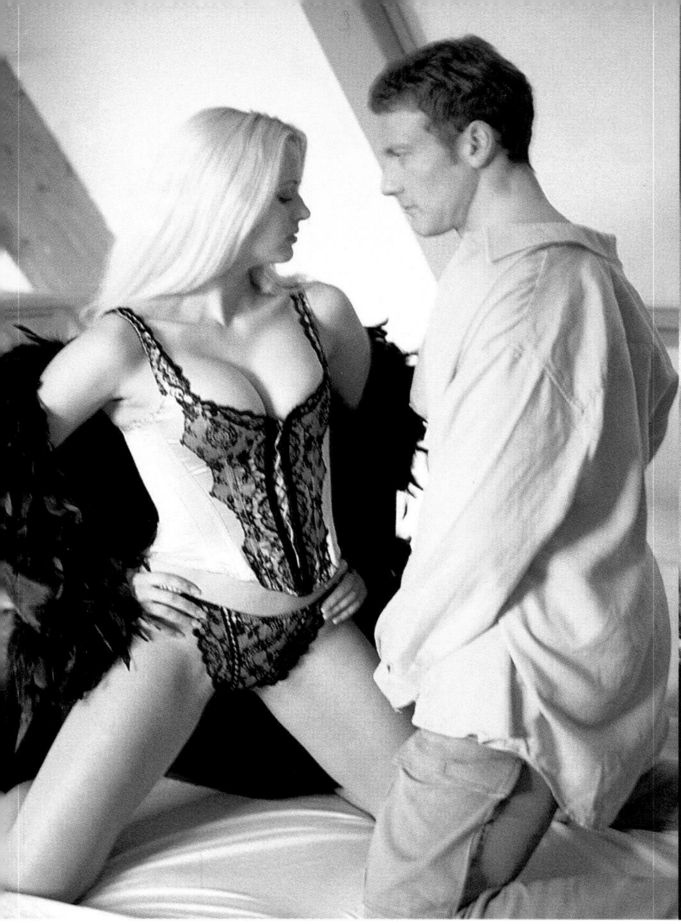

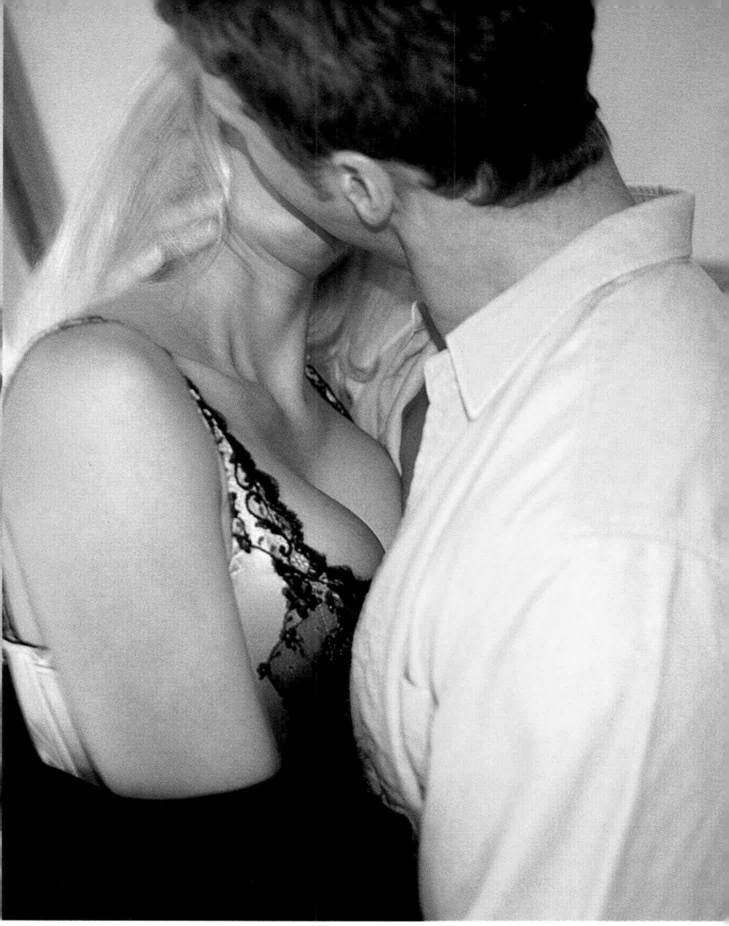

What bit of clothing makes you feel "There's no saying 'no' to me tonight"?

Plunging necklines, leather, velvet and anything tight and clingy are likely to do it for both sexes. High heels on women and large belt buckles on men often send an exceptionally sexual signal.

LOOKING SEXY

When you look at the sorts of clothes that put you in mind for sex you may soon find yourself straying into the bounds of fantasy. You can put a sparkle into your sex life by making sure that your ordinary clothing enhances your appearance and leads your thoughts to sex. But once you've the confidence to begin acknowledging what it is about your own or your partner's appearance that turns you on there may be other looks you would like to experiment with. What specific fantasy would you prefer to explore? Do you fancy the idea of a master/servant scenario which you and your partner can play out together? If so, consider

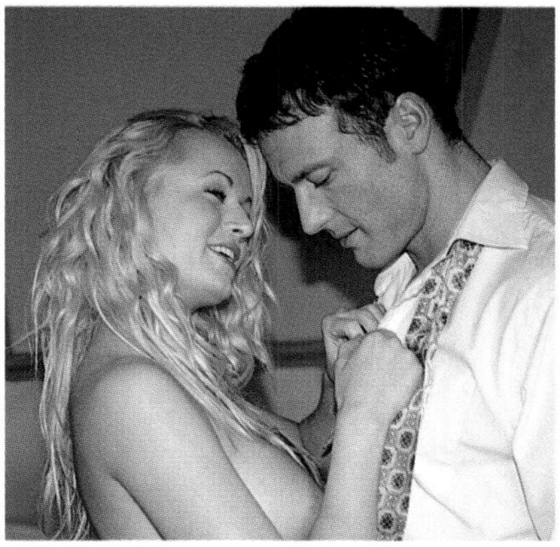

Dressing up with stripping off in mind

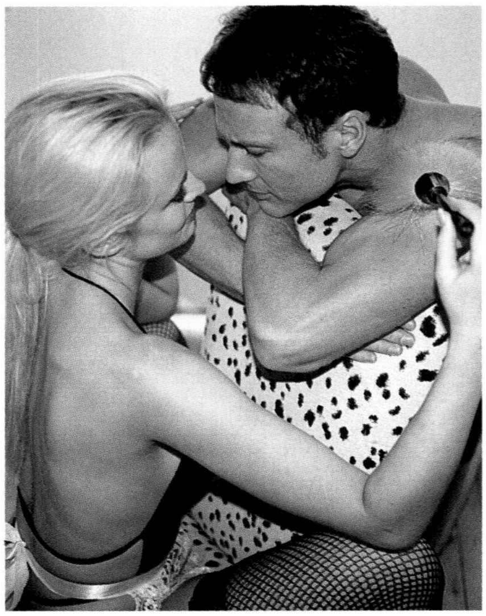

Feather dusters have more uses than tackling spiders

kitting one of you out as a French maid or a butler on call to the other. You'll need a short little black dress with a brief white apron, white collar and cuffs, black stockings and black shoes for her outfit. And, of course, a feather duster to sweep away those cobwebs and tickle his fancy. If he is to be the butler, he'll need a severe black suit and tie, white gloves and a tray on which he presents his mistress anything she demands – a cup of tea, a bottle of body oil, a feather or whip. Or you might like to pretend that one of you is the boss, the other the employee. You'll both need to be in sober business clothes but have the added surprise of very brief, very sexy underwear hiding under the black and grey. If the idea of this gets you going you can make believe you are making love on the boardroom table, sweeping aside business papers and diaries. Or how about one of you as a slave, the other an Arabian Nights' prince or princess calling for their favourite from the harem? The slave would have to be very briefly clad in a diaphanous costume made from transparent muslin or voile and the master or mistress in sumptuous silks and satins. One, especially sexy, article of clothing that many men and women find arousing is the corset. On the surface, there's little to recommend it. Corsets are tight and constricting, pulling the body into an exaggerated shape – which, of course, is the appeal. A corset gives its wearer an hourglass figure, pushing breasts into the open and making a waist look as if it can be spanned with one hand – an invitation to any spectator. They're also a challenge; wear one and you say "I'm so tightly trussed up. Can you cut my stays and unleash everything I'm holding back?" A slightly less extreme but no less sexy challenge is provided by the basque. This, too, is an

...black stockings and black shoes for her outfit. And, of course, a feather duster to sweep away those cobwebs and tickle his fancy.

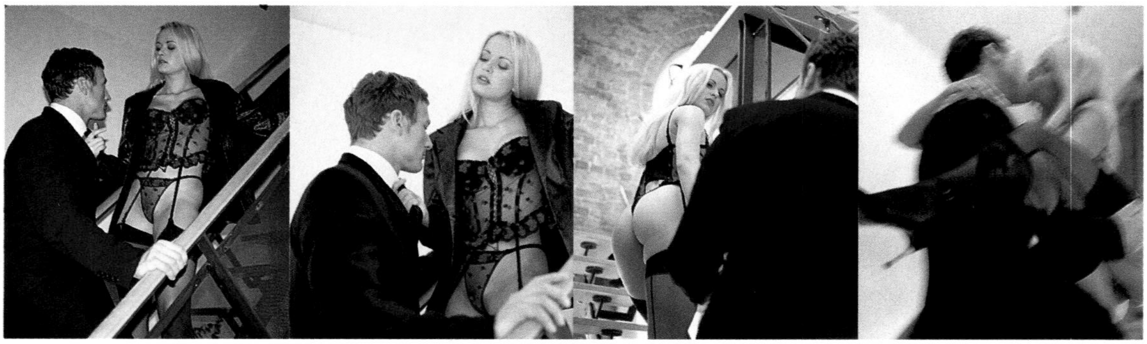

A severe suit can hide some surprises

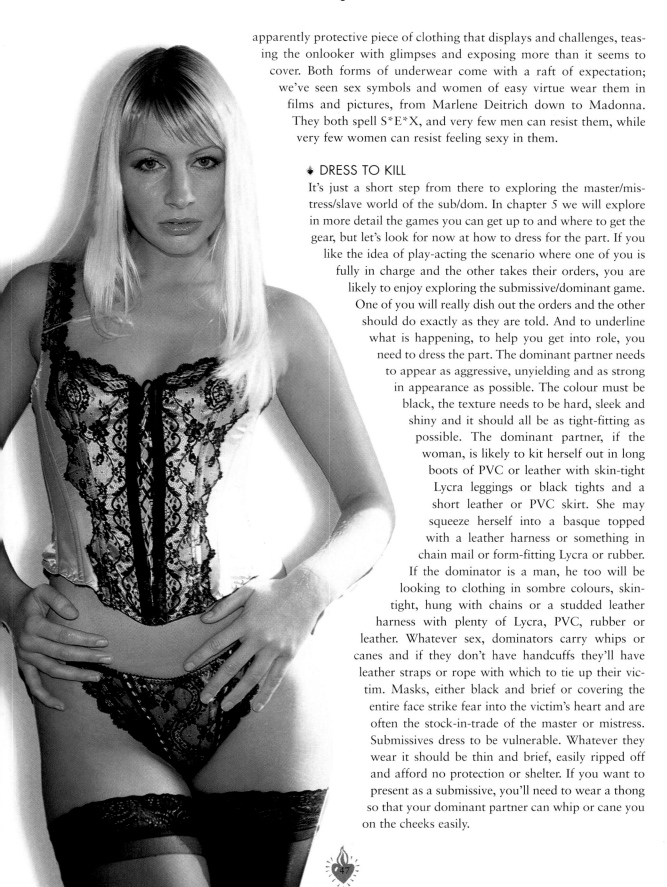

apparently protective piece of clothing that displays and challenges, teasing the onlooker with glimpses and exposing more than it seems to cover. Both forms of underwear come with a raft of expectation; we've seen sex symbols and women of easy virtue wear them in films and pictures, from Marlene Deitrich down to Madonna. They both spell S*E*X, and very few men can resist them, while very few women can resist feeling sexy in them.

DRESS TO KILL

It's just a short step from there to exploring the master/mistress/slave world of the sub/dom. In chapter 5 we will explore in more detail the games you can get up to and where to get the gear, but let's look for now at how to dress for the part. If you like the idea of play-acting the scenario where one of you is fully in charge and the other takes their orders, you are likely to enjoy exploring the submissive/dominant game. One of you will really dish out the orders and the other should do exactly as they are told. And to underline what is happening, to help you get into role, you need to dress the part. The dominant partner needs to appear as aggressive, unyielding and as strong in appearance as possible. The colour must be black, the texture needs to be hard, sleek and shiny and it should all be as tight-fitting as possible. The dominant partner, if the woman, is likely to kit herself out in long boots of PVC or leather with skin-tight Lycra leggings or black tights and a short leather or PVC skirt. She may squeeze herself into a basque topped with a leather harness or something in chain mail or form-fitting Lycra or rubber. If the dominator is a man, he too will be looking to clothing in sombre colours, skin-tight, hung with chains or a studded leather harness with plenty of Lycra, PVC, rubber or leather. Whatever sex, dominators carry whips or canes and if they don't have handcuffs they'll have leather straps or rope with which to tie up their victim. Masks, either black and brief or covering the entire face strike fear into the victim's heart and are often the stock-in-trade of the master or mistress. Submissives dress to be vulnerable. Whatever they wear it should be thin and brief, easily ripped off and afford no protection or shelter. If you want to present as a submissive, you'll need to wear a thong so that your dominant partner can whip or cane you on the cheeks easily.

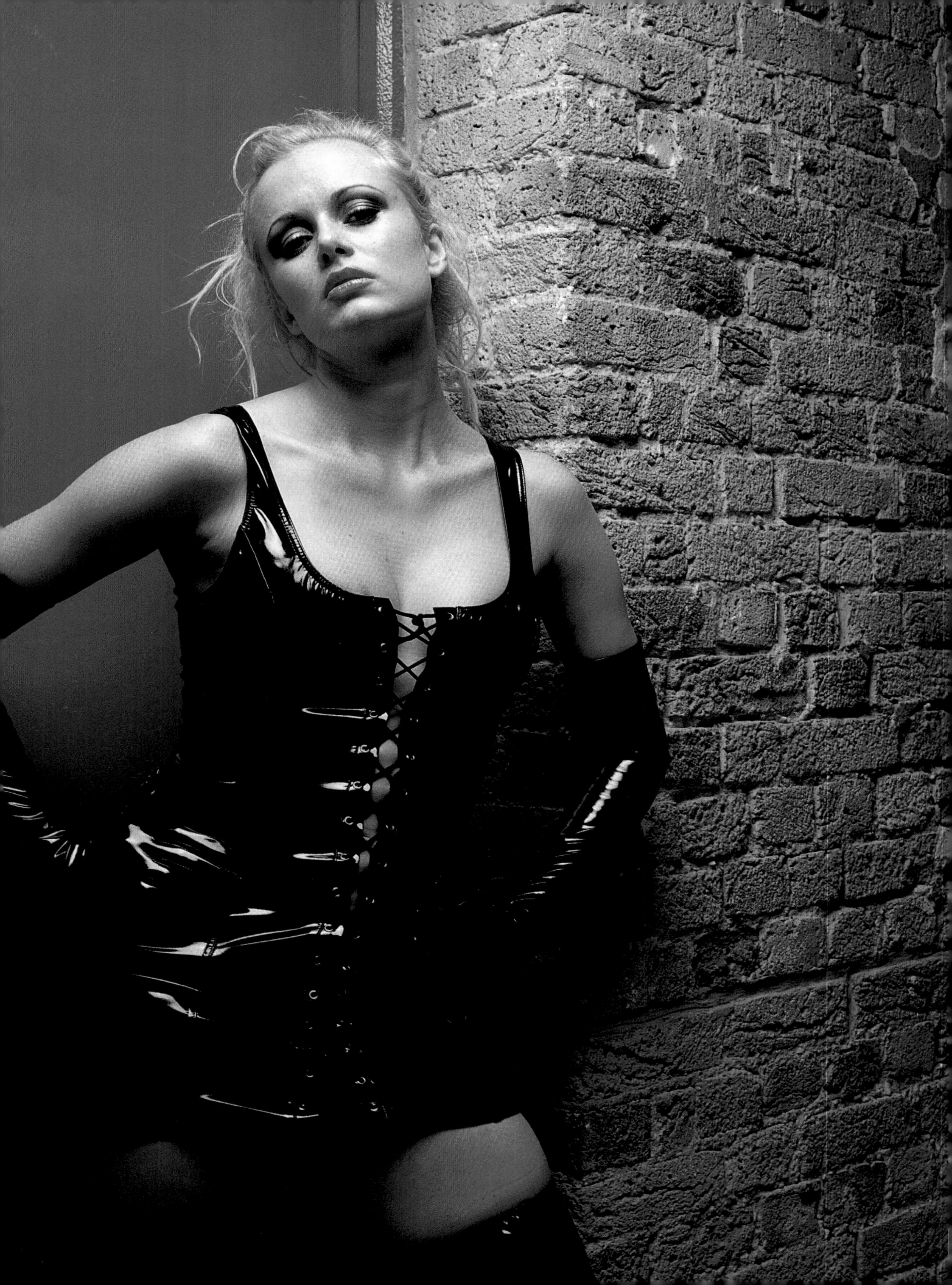

TRANSGENDER DRESSING

A final twist on dressing for sex may be experimenting with swapping clothes. Many men are turned on by the experience of her wearing the pants – his pants – and him wearing hers! Spend a hilarious hour kitting each other out in your favourite outfit and seeing how your partner looks wearing it. You could then discover exactly how easy – or difficult – it is for you to strip your partner down for sex, or for either of you to shrug out of your own clothing. Swapping clothes could be part of a fantasy scenario, with each of you exploring what it might be like to experience sex from the other side of the gender divide. You could play-act being the opposite sex, or simply feel what some of the difference may be. You may discover a new taste for transgender dressing. As we've said before, you'll never know until you try.

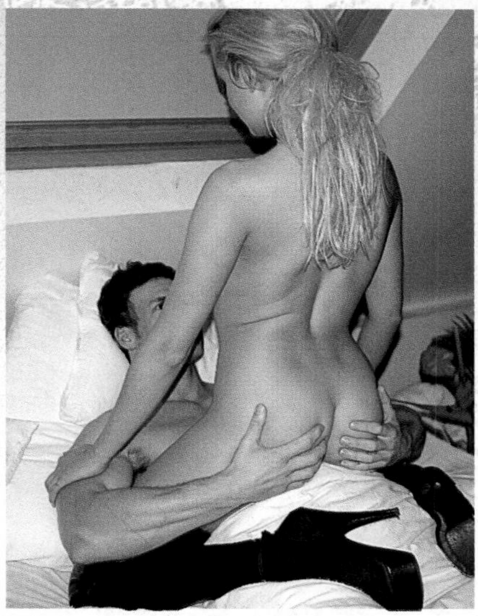

Sensual pleasure in rubber and leather

Clothes are an important way of enhancing your sex life together, the icing on the cake. There is no doubt that certain clothing or materials can become inextricably entwined with particular people's sexual desires. Many men, for instance, find the idea of high heels quite exciting. There are several explanations for this.

Whether he realizes it or not, a woman in high heels puts a man in mind of sex.

One is that high heels extend the line of the leg, pressing a certain instinctive button in our psyche. We are programmed to find certain survival traits attractive. Way back in the caveman days, any sensible man would want a mate who could have it away on her toes at speed at the approach of a dangerous predator. Long, shapely and muscular legs were a distinct advantage in a mate and a pair of high heels presents exactly that appearance. But there could be another and sexier reason. One of the reactions to orgasm in a woman is the so-called carpopedal reflex, when the toes curl and the foot straightens. Whether he realizes it or not, a woman in high heels puts a man in mind of sex. But for some men, high heels attain a fetishistic interest. Here the explanation might be that early experiences as a baby at their mother's feet quite literally fixes their interest and their reaction on her footwear. Similarly, both sexes can get aroused by the feel or scent of rubber or some other material if their first experiences of sensual pleasure was as babies wrapped up in such materials. If you find that certain things tickle your taste buds and have you reacting, why not pursue

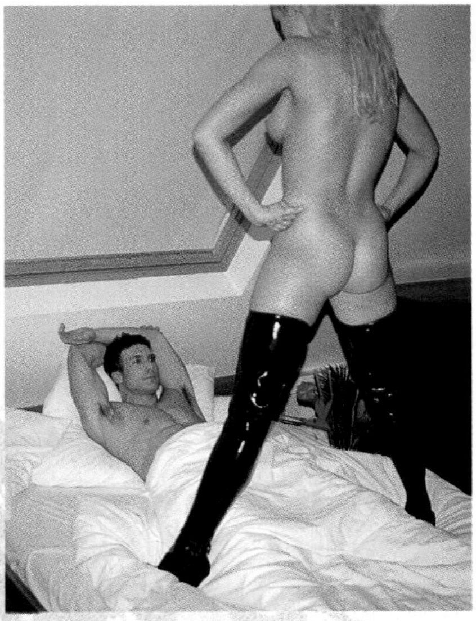

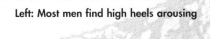

Left: Most men find high heels arousing

and explore this? There is, however, one warning. Few people mind a particular interest being catered for within a shared sex life when it's an extra and an enhancement. In other words, if high-heeled shoes help you see your partner as infinitely desirable and arousing, then it's an advantage. Trouble starts, not when you like to incorporate this extra, but when you can't do without it. If you find yourself preferring sex better with than without, or if indeed you don't like to or can't perform without it, then it's time to ask for help. Nobody likes to feel their partner is more in love with a pair of kitten heels than they are with them.

and both sexes would welcome such a display.

The key point to keep in mind is that every good strip needs tease. Stripping for sex is not just a question of getting your kit off. Think of birthdays and parcels. The more elaborate the packaging, the longer it takes to peel away the layers, the higher the anticipation and the greater the satisfaction. So start a strip fully clothed. If you want to go the whole hog, dim the lights and put some good bump-and-grind music on. "The Stripper" is an obvious tune but something like Joe Cocker's "You Can Keep Your Hat On" is even better. Put on extras – a hat, gloves, a scarf or tie – even if you never normally wear them. The longer

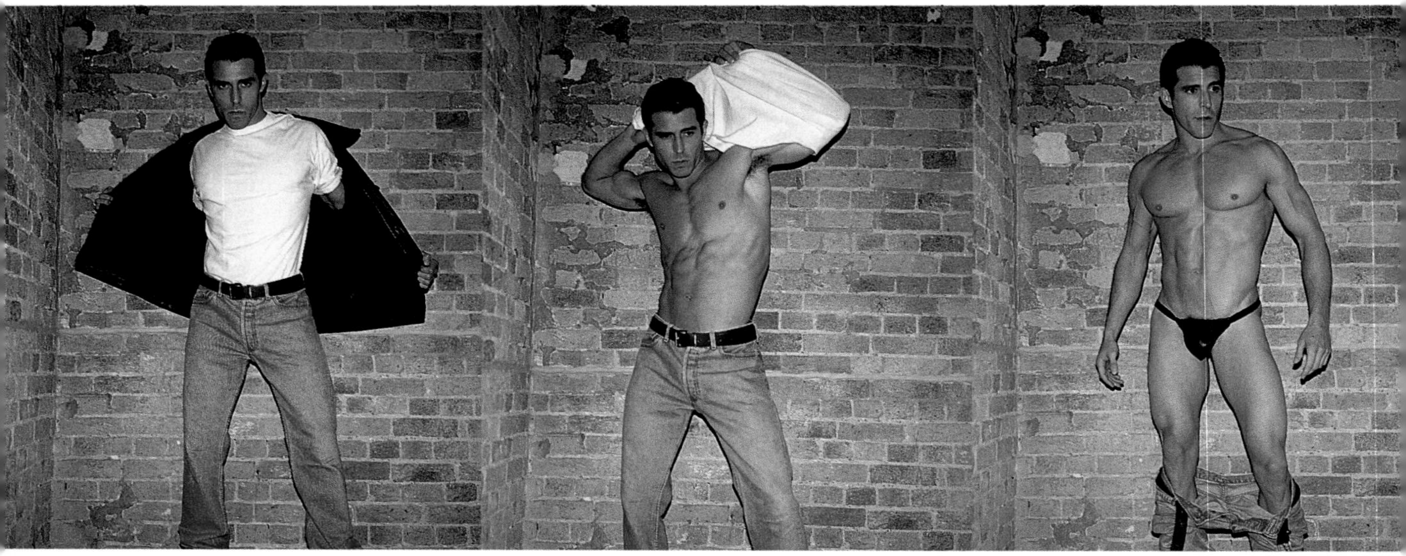

Few women can resist their man doing a "Full Monty"

GETTING YOUR KIT OFF

Did Adam and Eve really cover their nakedness for shame? Or did they add to their original sins by being the first to realize that concealing parts of the body can be far more erotic, suggestive and exciting than letting everything hang out? Putting on the right clothes to put yourself or your partner in the mood is one element of dressing for sex. Another is knowing how to take them off. There are times when simply ripping off your clothes and those of your partner and falling on to the floor, bed or kitchen table is just what you need and want. But doing a striptease for your partner has its merits

it takes to get you down to your thong, the greater frenzy you'll be working your audience into! Peel off an item at a time remembering that you never want to look foolish. Depending on your tastes, men tend to look better if they take off shoes and socks first while most men get a kick out of seeing her shoes and stockings left on until quite late in the proceedings. A lot of men and women find incongruity quite arousing, so leaving a hat on until last or removing a shirt before a tie can have its appeal. Move to the music, and wrap each item you remove around yourself, or drag it between your legs as if you're pleasuring yourself with it, before discarding it. Invite your audience

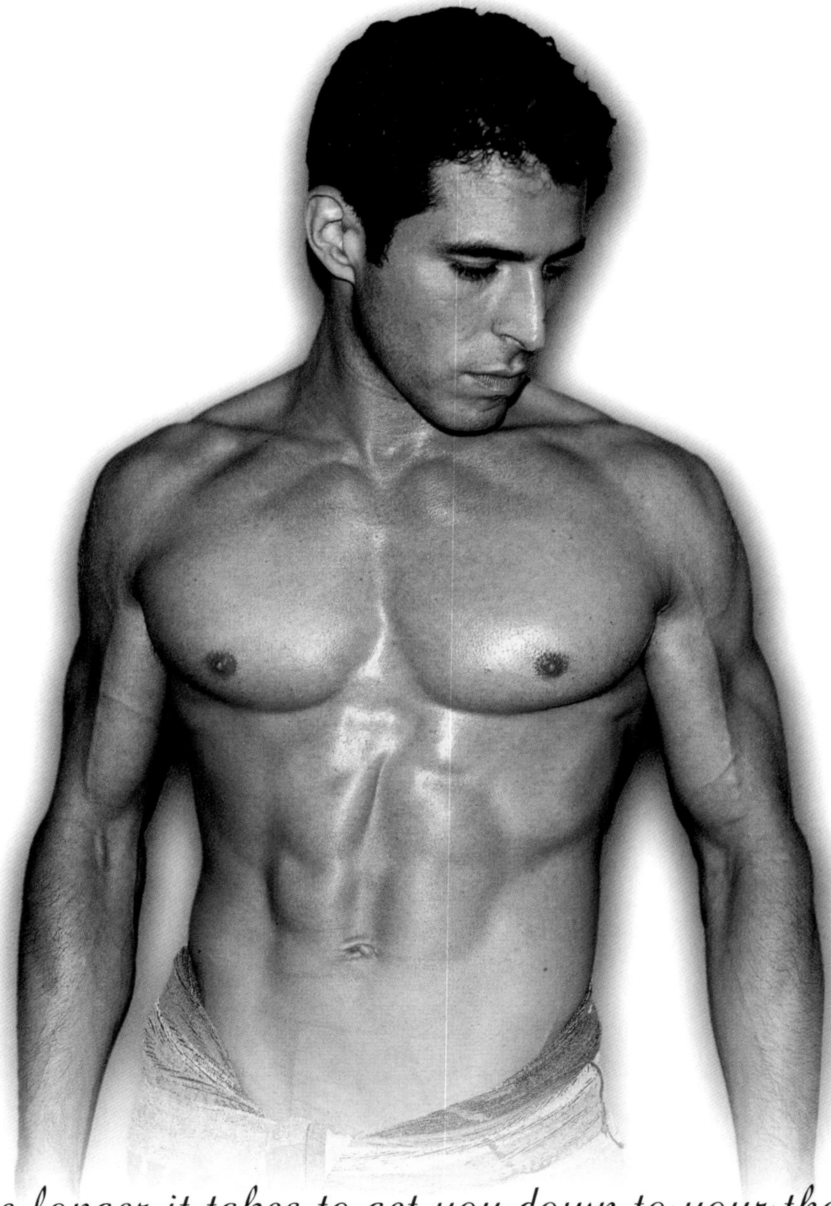

The longer it takes to get you down to your thong, the greater frenzy you'll be working your audience into!

to participate, removing a vital garment with their teeth, for instance, or holding a belt or tie as you unravel it from around yourself. Strut in front of your partner, coming close to tempt them but then retreating to make love to a lampshade, door or armchair instead of them. When you're finally down to one scrap of clothing, invite them to smooth talcum powder or oil all over you, before finally putting them out of their misery by removing the last item and concealing yourself behind a hat, scarf or fan.

Seeing a partner take off their clothes in a sexy and inviting way is a delight shared by almost everyone and a virtually guaranteed turn-on. Even if you don't want to go to the length of a formal striptease, you can at least abide by "good stripping rules" and get your clothes off in a way that is not going to turn your bed partner frigid at the sight. Basically, the prime rule of kit removal for both sexes is to think about what comes off, what stays on and how you will look as you do it. What is vitally important in all this is the actual order in which you do things. As has already been mentioned, the most common and libido-reducing mistake for a man is to leave the socks on to the bitter end. It then becomes the ultimate turn-off if the socks happen to be black, dark-coloured or jokey. So if, for some bizarre reason, you can't break yourself out of the socks-last habit, at least buy yourself some socks of the slightly less ridiculous white or light-coloured variety. In fact, pairing some sporty-looking briefs with white socks is quite a turn on, and not only for gay men!

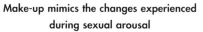

Make-up mimics the changes experienced during sexual arousal

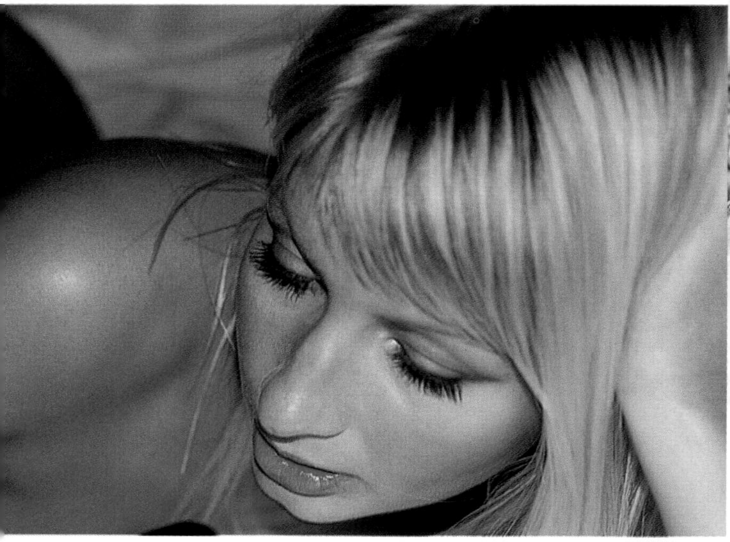

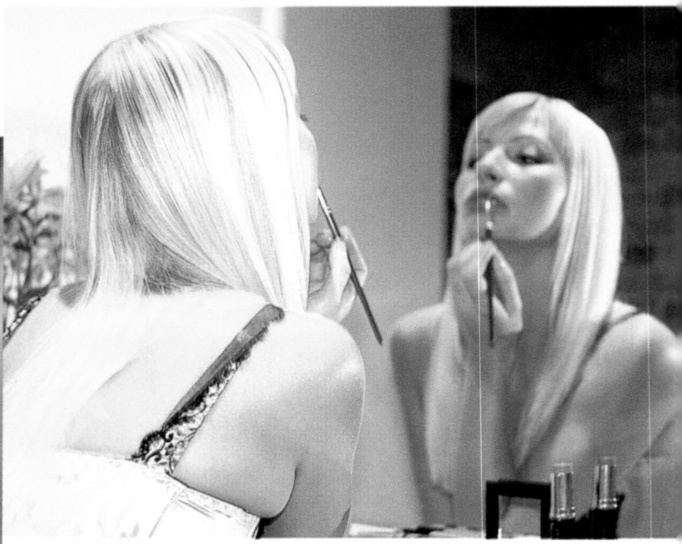

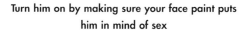

Turn him on by making sure your face paint puts him in mind of sex

CROWNING GLORY

When you're dressing for sex, don't forget your own natural assets. The fact that most puritan cultures insist on a woman covering her hair tells you that, whether on the head or on the body, it is an intensely sexy part of our bodies, and is so for both sexes. Some women are turned on by male facial hair, some are turned off. Talk about it and find out which one your partner prefers. A few days shadow could do wonders for your sex life! But think about body hair, too. Some women find the idea of a smooth, tanned, oiled chest drives them wild. If so, make with the razor or better still, the depilatory cream. Waxing would, of course, show total dedication and be mucho macho. Do it at home or have it done for you, smooth on the oil and *voila*! Most men say they love their partners to have long hair, but if that's not your style confuse them by directing their attention elsewhere. Female body hair is supposed to be unattractive, with overtones of masculinity. More significantly, it has animalistic overtones, and since you want to bring out the tiger in him, you may find leaving your armpits unshaved for a time has the desirable effect. You could also consider a new form of hair dressing: pubic hair. Some men go wild at the sight of shaved genitals. Others would be aroused by a small touch, such as using clippers and a razor to turn your pubic hair to a heart by shaping the top line. In fact, women may also be aroused by the sight of denuded, shaved genitals. While removing the fuzz on a woman has the effect of taking her back to a pre-pubertal look, in men it is more likely to emphasize size – he can seem larger, the barer he is.

Make-up also has a particular impact when you're planning a look that invites your partner to have sex. Cosmetics have been in use for as long as five thousand years. Every society we can find has tried its own methods of improving on nature in this way. The early Greeks, for example, used white lead, antimony and seaweed extracts, while Roman women put on ground deer antlers and honey. In ancient Egypt, women even had special cushions to rest their elbows on to guarantee the steadiest of paint jobs.

PAINTING BY NUMBERS

As well as their function in gilding the lily, cosmetics have an equally long history of being used as indicators of the wearer's sexual intentions. It might unsettle you to know that wearing bright red lipstick in Nero's Rome was a form of advertising. You would have been saying that your particular speciality was oral sex. Most people are quite unaware of the real reason we darken our eyelids, redden our lips and apply blusher to cheeks. If you thought it was just to make you look pretty, think again. Look at yourself in the mirror next time you are aroused, and you'll see the real motive. When you become sexually excited, several changes take place over your body, and in your face. Your pupils enlarge, making your eyes appear larger and darker. Your face flushes, bringing colour to your cheeks and making the lips and the lobes of your ears redden and swell. Indeed, the addition of perfume copies the body scent your partner would notice on your heated body. Make-up is attractive, not only because it makes its wearer appear sexually aroused, but because it makes the viewer aroused too. This is because looking at a person who seems aroused by you is the biggest turn-on possible. If you want to use your make-up to effect, look at yourself in the mirror when excited and then copy the signs you see. Try it on places other than the obvious; use colour on your nipples, the ear lobes and inside of the nostrils and your chest to tell your partner they've got you all hot and bothered.

> *When you become sexually excited, several changes take place over your body, and in your face. When you apply make-up, you mimic exactly these changes.*

We're not being excluding or sexist here, either. This advice may sound all very "women only", but remember that male sexual arousal creates exactly the same physical signs and that a skilful use of make-up can also work its wonders for him too. Beauty preparations have always been used by men as much as by women. Nero was renowned for his liberal use of eye shadow and the *Kama Sutra*, in describing the morning ritual of the average citizen, suggests he "apply a limited quantity of ointments and perfumes to his body, put collyrium on his eyelids and below his eyes and colour his lips with alacktaka". In the eighteenth and nineteenth centuries, powdered periwigs and scented handkerchiefs were hardly the sole preserve of the ladies. Far from emasculating men, the use of adornment allowed the peacock to strut his stuff and proclaim his sexual interests as much as the peahen. And don't forget perfume when dressing for sex. Remember Marilyn Monroe, who when asked what she wore in bed said, "Chanel No.5." Cologne, whether perfume or aftershave, can add to the turn-on, and the best way to find the one that will have the desired effect is to ask your partner to choose yours. Since you want them to be aroused by it, they should pick it – and you're likely to find that the one they want is the scent that comes nearest to mimicking your body smell when aroused. Smelling, however expensively, of a summer meadow or sea spray might not get the result you actually want.

You would probably get better results by letting Nature take its course and forgetting about buying perfumes altogether. Sweat may sound nasty and not seem to be the obvious first choice as a turn-on, but mixed in with the one-and-a-half pints the

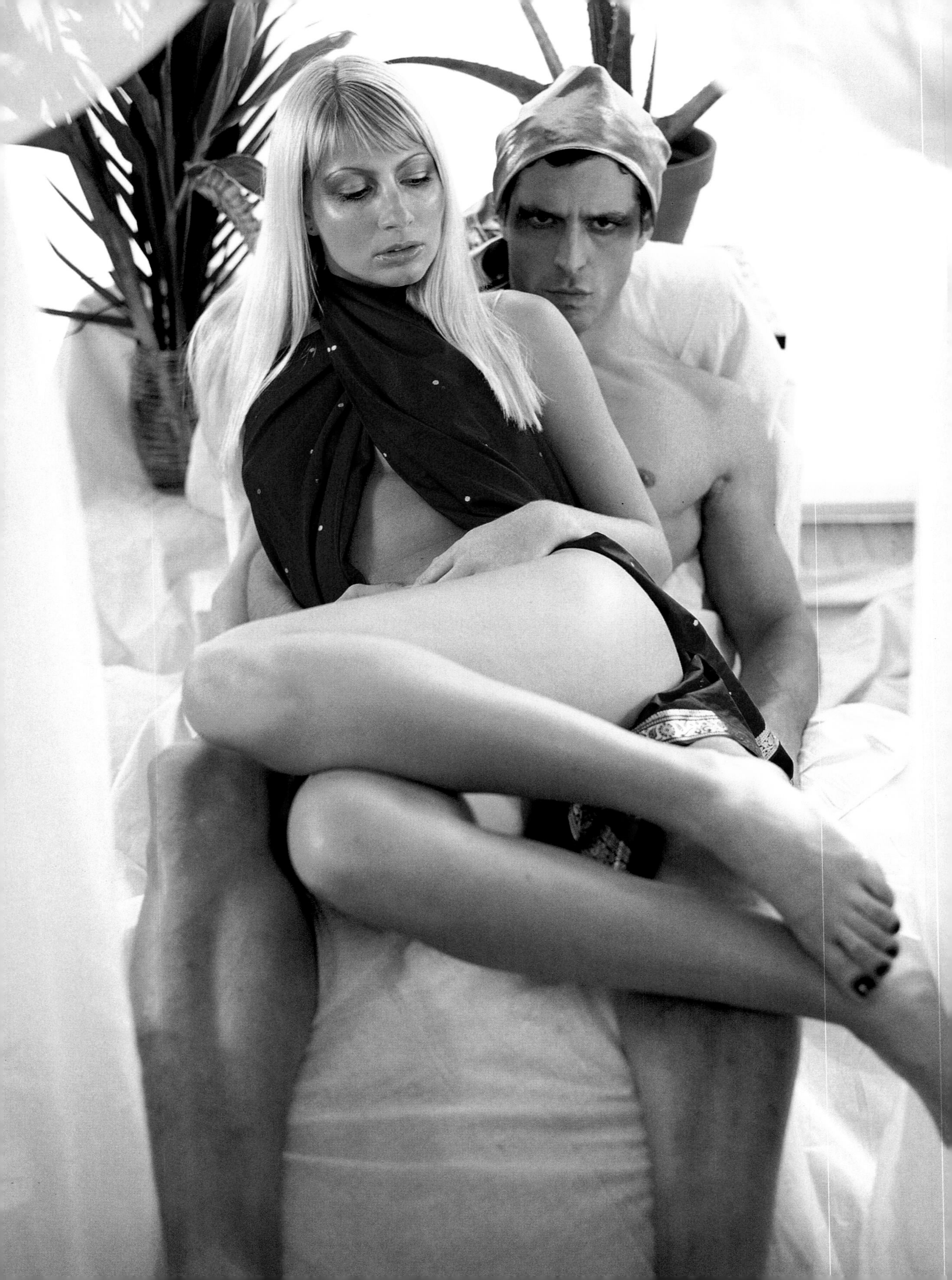

average body produces each day are chemical substances called pheromones, which send out sexy signals to potential lovers. So try a freebie to attract yours. Stay fresh – it's stale sweat that is offensive – but stop masking those pheromones with deodorants, perfumes and aftershave. The smell of the real you should have far more appeal than anything you can get out of an expensive bottle.

Cosmetics are temporary and changeable, but how about a tattoo as a more permanent adornment for your biggest organ – the seventeen square feet of skin that covers the average body? You could find that a well-drawn and strategically-placed tattoo could be one of the most erotic ways you could adorn your body. A butterfly or bird on a buttock or hip or just above the pubic hairline, placed where it can only be seen when you're naked, can be intensely exciting. If you do decide to have one done, make doubly sure that your tattooist is reputable and practises a strict code of hygiene. And do recognize that the result is permanent and that even modern laser technology cannot remove the signs of a tattoo completely. Once you have decided on your design, it's yours for life, so do start small!

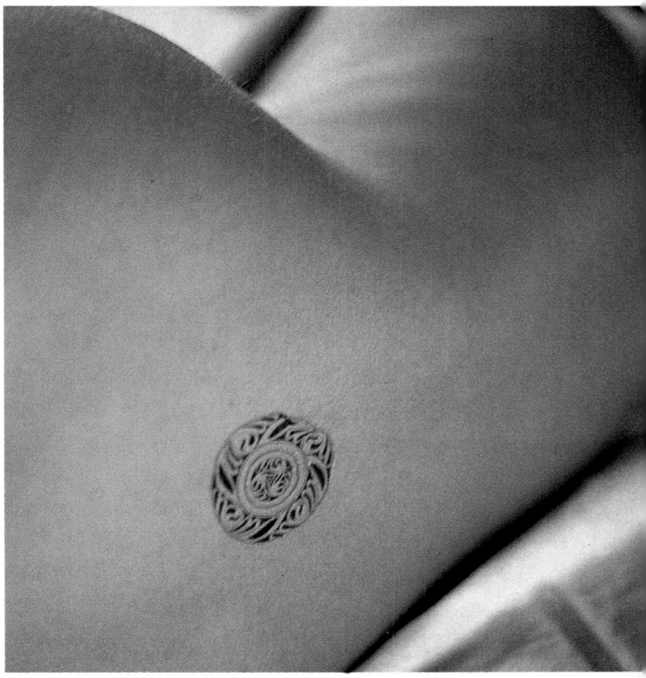

Body art draws the eye and says "For your secret enjoyment"

Cosmetics are temporary and changeable, but how about a tattoo as a more permanent adornment for your biggest organ - the seventeen square feet of skin that covers the average body?

BODY ART

Another form of body art that dresses us up and appeals to a partner to undress us is jewellery. We wear earrings to draw attention to a sexually sensitive area, the ear lobes. These are rich in nerve endings and many people can be brought to a pitch of sensual awareness by having them nibbled or sucked or blown on. Many men find earrings erotic for that reason – the longer and more elaborate and dangling the better. Gently sucking at, flicking or tugging on an earring can have dramatic effects on its owner. But why not consider piercing other, more sensitive, areas when you think about dressing for sex? Rings and studs through the eyebrow, nose and belly button may now be considered old hat, having moved from extreme to High Street fashion. But what about piercings through the nipple, foreskin (male or female), penis or clitoris, labia or scrotum? Sounds extreme, but wearers say it sensitizes the area dramatically and they can be brought to full arousal and even orgasm, by themselves or partner, by gently manipulating the ring or stud. Men and women also say that a strategically placed stud in their own genitals can be used to drive their partner wild when making love.

Left: Adorn your body with sumptuous fabrics, jewellery and make-up to get you in the mood

GET FIT

If you feel that your body needs a little more than just clothing or make-up, tattooing or piercing to adorn it sufficiently, you can always think about improving it by sensible eating and exercise. If, though, you want an effect that can't be given by any amount of fresh fruit or sweaty hours in the gym you can bring at least your clothes' appearance nearer to your ideal by judicious choice of underwear. Strait-lacing and boned corsets may now be only the specialist preserve of those with this particular fetish, but modern materials such as nylon and Lycra can be used to obtain the silhouette you crave without putting your internal organs at risk.

At the furthest extreme on the road to the body beautiful is the knife and the other tools of the cosmetic surgeon's trade. There would seem to be no limit other than the amount you can afford to have medical skill re-shape your body. Faces can be lifted, noses and ears can be altered, bottoms tightened and even the genitals can be "tidied up". Breast size can be increased. This is usually done by implanting a bag of silicone in between the pectoral muscle and the breast tissue, pushing out the owner's own natural assets. Such an operation is supposed to have no effect on the woman's ability to feel sensation but any of her lovers might find the new sight better than its touch. It may look good from a distance, but some men who have partners who have had a little too much added to their measurements describe making love to them as being like trying to enjoy yourself while lying on a concrete ramp! Surgeons can take away just as easily as they can add. Breasts, and many other parts of the body, can be reduced in size if that's what is wanted. One method of achieving this type of body shaping is liposuction – the "vacuuming" of unwanted fat from hips, thighs and elsewhere.

Cosmetic surgery might seem to be the magic wand that cures all bodily ills and dissatisfactions, but it has its own downside. Altering the part of your body that you might have convinced yourself is the only reason for shyness, embarrassment or any sexual disappointments will not necessarily remove them. If you dislike your body and feel lacking in self-esteem and self-confidence, altering a nose or breast may leave you still feeling inadequate and unattractive, but considerably poorer and bruised. And the process of looking for the wand can put you firmly and dangerously in the land of the medical cowboy. Unbelievably, a doctor in the UK does not have to have any specialist qualifications to practise cosmetic surgery and there are sadly practitioners and clinics who are far more interested in your money than in your physical or emotional well-being. The only safe away to approach cosmetic surgery (after taking counselling or giving considerable thought as to whether this is really for you) is by referral to a reputable surgeon or clinic through your own family doctor.

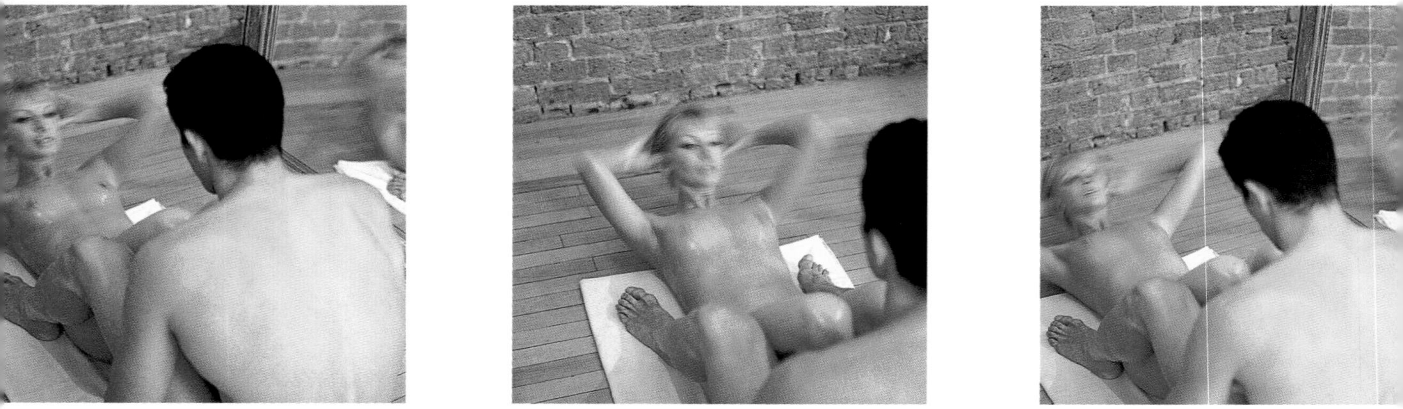

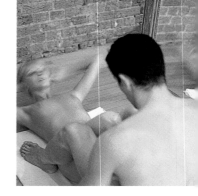

Personal training can get very personal

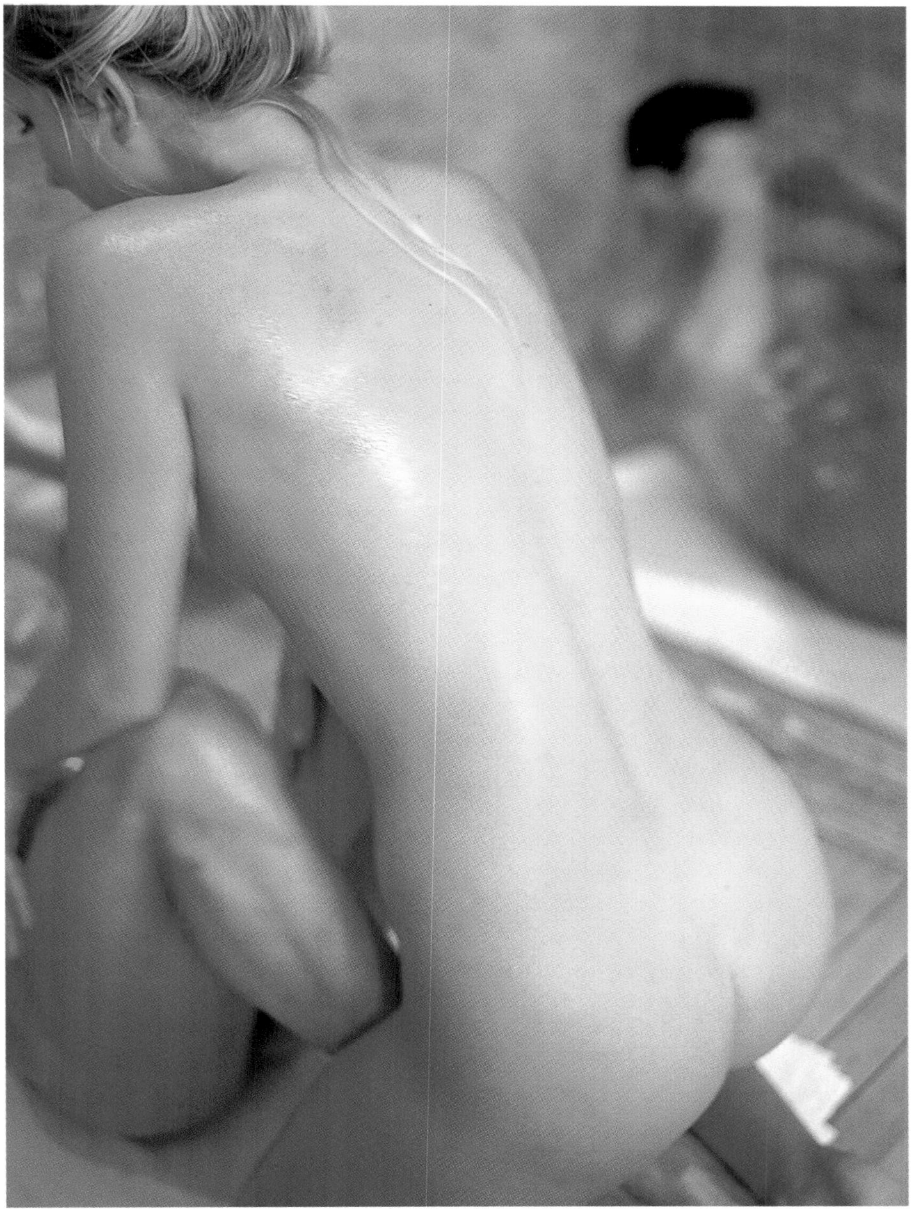

If you feel that your body needs a little more than just clothing or make-up, tattooing or piercing to adorn it sufficiently, you can always think about improving it by sensible eating and exercise.

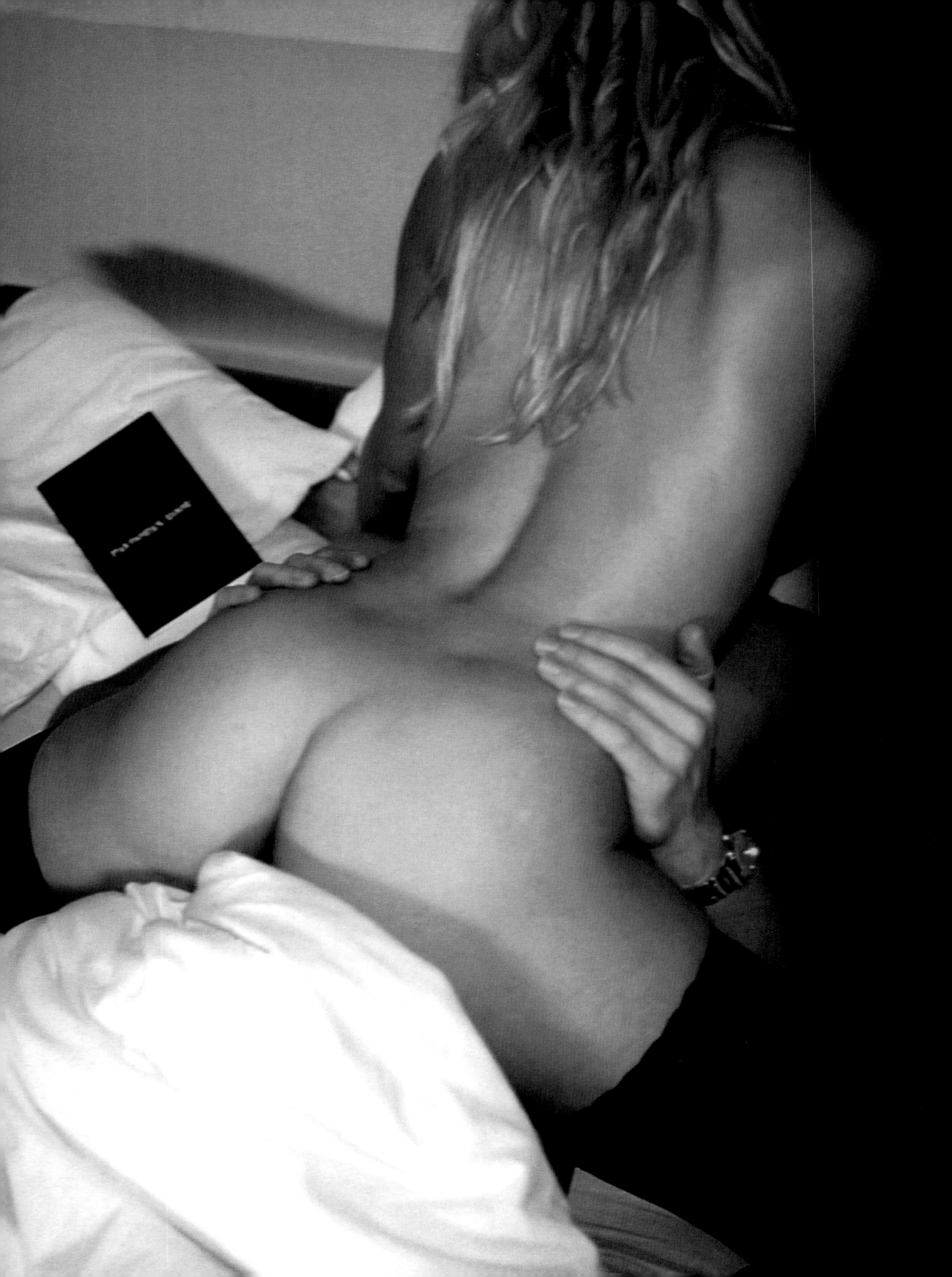

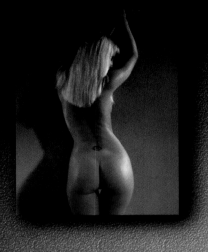

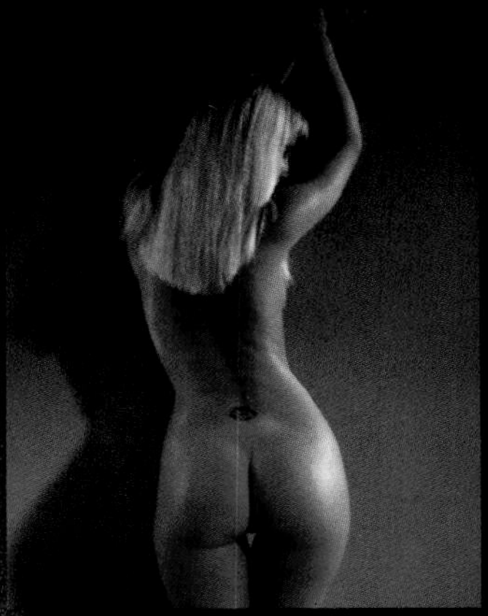

Chapter 4

PLAY TIME

You can experiment in sex and experience a wide range of sexual variation on many levels. You don't need to try anything outlandish to be new and different, simply turning the lights down low and lighting a candle or two will do it. But many people do want to try additions to their love life, and sex toys are the most obvious, widespread and easily obtained and used.

We are often fascinated but rather alarmed by the subject of sex toys, especially the sort of equipment that seems to come only from sex shops or mail order firms. But, let's face it, we're fascinated and sometimes alarmed by the subject of sex. This means we're primed to be enthralled by anything that may add pleasure, diversity and a touch of extra spice to our sex lives. Anyone can, and many people do, use sex toys to liven up their love lives and give pleasure to themselves and their partners.

Sex toys come with a history that stretches back hundreds and perhaps even thousands of years, and across cultures. The ancient Babylonians, Greeks and Japanese left paintings and text that showed how to make and use penis-substitutes, made from ivory, wood, glass or even carrots. These were called dildoes, which is still the term for a penis-shaped sex toy that isn't driven with power – although, confusingly, some companies marketing sex toys offer power driven ones as well. There are plenty of present day devices that can help you expand your love life, from vibrators to love eggs, Thai beads to "stud creams", penis rings to vacuum pumps.

Vibrators are probably the best known form of sex toy. Vibrators use battery or mains power to make them buzz and tremble rhythmically. Held against the body, they are stimulating and arousing for both sexes. Some are shaped like a penis and can be anything from the slim-line, at five inches long with a diameter of about one inch, to seven inches long and two inches around. Some are smooth, made of hard plastic or with a metallic finish. Others are grooved, with ribbing or bumps. And some are covered in soft latex to give a fleshy, warm and softer texture with authentic-looking veins. The newest material is a form of plastic or latex that manufacturers refer to as "jelly". It's soft, comes in a range of realistic-looking colours and textures and is just hard enough to have an effect without being so unyielding as to hurt. Just like the real thing in fact.

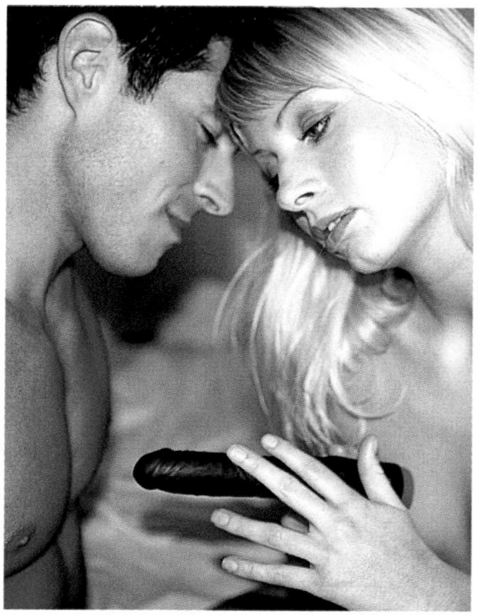

All-round fun for both sexes

Some penis-shaped vibrators have extra knobs or projections around the base, designed to give special attention to the clitoris. On some, these are just bumps or ribs. On others, these are extended finger-like extensions, designed to reach some way. For fun, many are shaped like animals, such as penguins, bears, kangaroos and koalas – or even people. Some vibrators have a distinct bend at the end. These are supposed to touch and stimulate the G-Spot, an area on the upper wall and some two-thirds along the vagina. When excited, this is reputed to provoke powerful orgasms and a burst of fluid known as female ejaculate. Other types of vibrators have a double end – one for the vagina or sex passage and the other for the rectum or back passage. Penis-shaped vibrators can tremble but may also rotate or move from side to side, or both. Some even have a reservoir that can be filled with warm liquid, to squirt out as a convincing ejaculation.

PADS AND EGGS

Not all vibrators are penis-shaped. Some resemble an oblong pad, designed to fit against the vulva, pressing against the clitoris and vagina. Some are shaped like small eggs. Also available are vibrating tongues. These not only vibrate, but also twist around so that for couples who really enjoy oral sex, but are flagging in the tongue area, this can come to the rescue. Penis-shaped vibrators in particular are designed with the intention of being used to stimulate women, though of course if anything can be seen as "gender free" it's sexual pleasure. But there are two designs made with men in mind. One is a small

You can use them on your own, to find out just what does turn you on. Or you can use them with a partner, with each person stimulating themselves or the other.

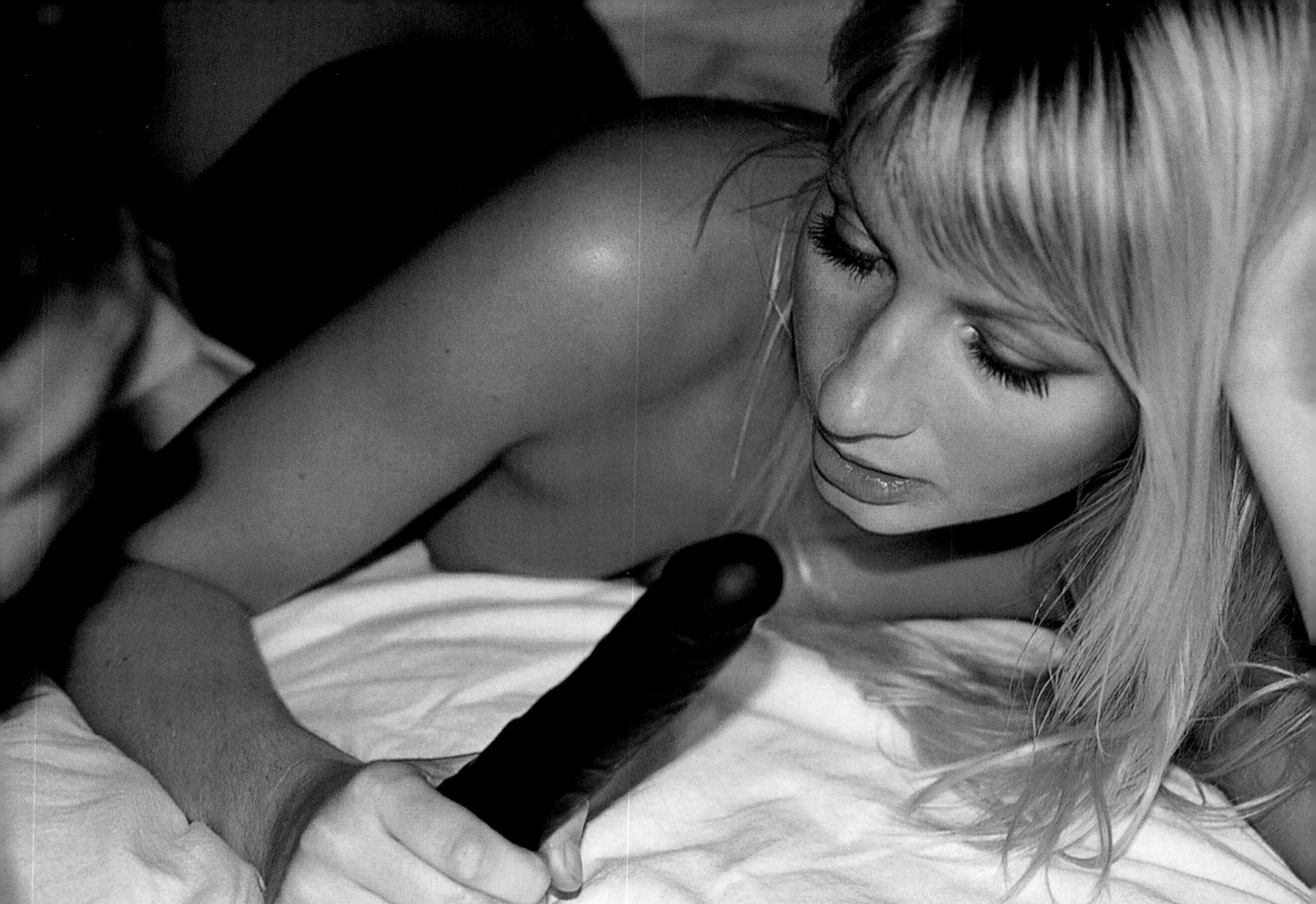

lozenge-shaped device fastened to a ring, that you attach to the penis. The small buzzing device is then held against the shaft or under the penis and against the scrotum. And the other is an artificial vagina. These are latex or rubber tubes, with a realistic appearance, lined with smooth latex or soft projections.

There are other vibrators that are widely available, but which are marketed as having other uses. You can buy a massager that is advertised as being for the relief of tension as well as muscular aches and pains and stiffness. The inference is that you use it to massage your neck, shoulders or feet. It certainly relieves tension, but not perhaps in the way its manufacturers might like you to think they recommend! This device looks a bit like a hair dryer. They usually come with a variety of attachments that fit on the business end, in a range of bumps, lumps and twiddly bits.

So how do vibrators work and what do you do with them? The vibrations, when pressed against the body, are highly stimulating. Some have a steady speed, from slow to fast. Some can be adjusted to go from a slow and gentle tremor to full-scale throbbing. You can use them on your own, to find out just what does turn you on. Or you can use them with a partner, with each person stimulating themselves or the other. When you read many of the catalogues from firms that sell vibrators, the suggestion seems to be that vibrators are mainly used to arouse women, and by operating them as a penis substitute, inside the vagina. As more and more people are discovering and realizing, you don't even have to use a penis internally, in penetrative sex, to enjoy it. In exactly the same way, vibrator users soon discover that this is not the main way of getting pleasure from a sex toy.

Vibrators are enormous fun. If you are going to use one as a penis, you may find it becomes even more stimulating if you use a cream or jelly for lubrication. They are particularly helpful in allowing partners to discover what sort of touches, in which particular places, really ring their bells. They have a particular place in the love life of anyone with any form of physical difficulty. If you have any sort of illness or disability that makes movement a problem or slows down sex, using a vibrator can bring friction and rhythm. But you don't have to have a difficulty to get full value from using such a sex toy.

GET BUZZING

If you'd like to try out a vibrator, first decide which type. The pad type are excellent if you want to be on your own and have your hands free to stimulate other parts of your body as well as your clitoris. A ring and lozenge can be used to arouse a male partner and also during sex. Then, they not only stimulate a man but, by making his penis thrum, can be highly exciting for his partner too. Penis-shaped vibrators are probably the best all-round fun and can be used by both sexes.

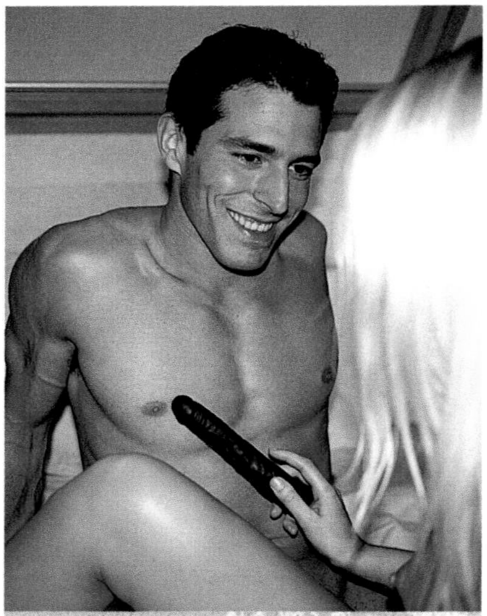

Make sure you are warm and comfortable and can't be overheard or interrupted.

Make sure you are warm and comfortable and can't be overheard or interrupted. Start with a gentle, buzzing speed. Run the vibrator over your body, touching your genitals and nipples briefly but concentrating at this point on everything else. Use the vibrator as you would your own or your partner's hand, just stroking up the inside of your legs and arms and down the outside, over your back, stomach and chest. Then do the same to your partner. Then, hand the vibrator to your partner and have them do the same, first to themselves and then you. Increase the speed and do it again, paying more attention to the bits you've found you liked having touched. Now concentrate on the more obvious excitable spots. Press the device against nipples, ear lobes, lips, neck and insides of elbows and knees. Finally, concentrate on clitoris and labia or penis and scrotum. Both partners may also find it stimulating to use the vibrations to stimulate around the back passage. If yours is a vibrator that specifies you can use it in water, try these exercises in the bath or shower, using soap to make you extra slippery. Or use lubricating jelly or cream to add a gliding sensation. Women are likely to find the most exciting and stimulating area is around the labia and clitoris, while men may find the best spots are the shaft of the penis and around the head or glans. But we are all individuals and you will find you have your own favourite bits, and they may not be the most obvious or common ones. The trick is to experiment, on your own or with a partner, to find out.

SAFER SEX

A few warnings. Don't use a vibrator anywhere near water, unless the instructions specifically say you can. Don't forget to have spare batteries on hand; there's nothing quite as frustrating, literally, as running flat at that critical moment. If you thought a three-year-old with a new toy on Christmas morning could hold the world record for screaming when discovering batteries are not included, wait till you hear a thirty-year-old with a flat vibrator! Do take the batteries out when travelling. Custom officers are very used to buzzing bags and red-faced passengers but you may find it embarrassing. Mind you, there's no point in feeling shy or humiliated. If anyone recognized the sound, it means they have one too, so who's to mock ?

Hygiene is important with vibrators. If you are sharing sex toys with anyone, consider using a condom. If there is any risk either of you has a sexual infection, this becomes a must. Even if you are certain of your infection status, remember that conditions such as thrush, while not being sexual diseases, are sexually

We are all individuals and you will find you have your own favourite bits, and they may not be the most obvious or common ones. The trick is to experiment, on your own or with a partner, to find out.

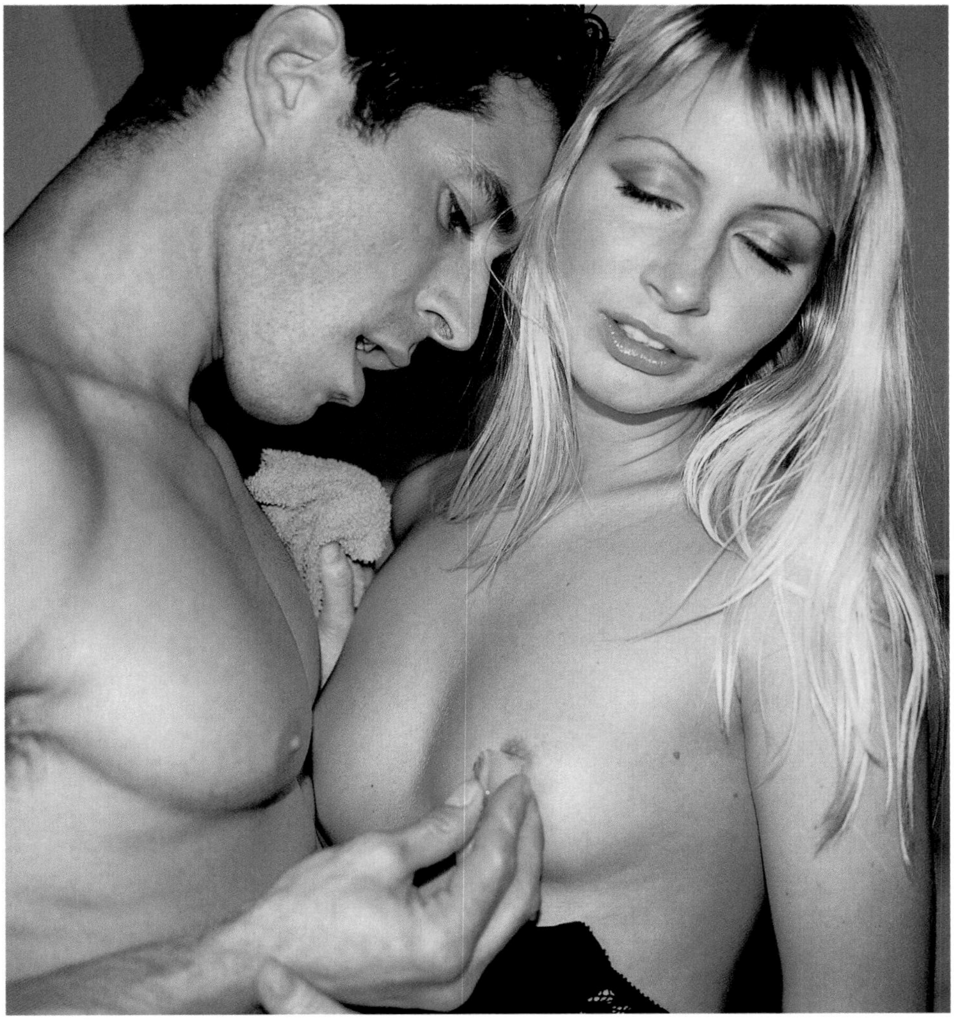

Vibrators and other sex toys, even ice cubes, can help you discover what you like

transmissible. Men often do not suffer thrush symptoms but can carry the bugs. It's not uncommon for women to suffer frequent attacks of thrush they find hard to treat. What is often happening is that they are beating their own infection only to have it passed back again when they next have sex with a partner who, because he doesn't have symptoms, doesn't realize he too is infected. But infection aside, vibrators can pass on nasties if you are experimenting with anal sex or it is part of your sexual repertoire. Organisms that thrive happily and healthily in the back passage can cause problems if carried to a woman's vagina or the water passage of either men or women. So even if you are using a vibrator on yourself and have no sexual infections, you can still give yourself an unpleasant infection if you use a vibrator in your own rectum and then place it in your own vagina, without either first cleaning it or putting on a fresh condom.

DONT GET LOST

You also have to be careful about what you put in the passages of your body. You can't "lose" a vibrator in the vagina. The actual entrance to the uterus or womb is very small and tightly closed. It is also offset, lying about two thirds of the way inside the vagina, on the upper wall. But it is possible to have an object become wedged inside the sex passage. When a woman becomes sexually aroused, the upper two-thirds of the sex passage widens and balloons out. It sets up a surprisingly strong inward pull. The greater the arousal, the greater the inward suction. Anything small that isn't attached to an outside source, such as a penis to its owner, can be pulled into the vagina and lodged behind the pubic bone when the woman has climaxed and relaxed. This is why it can be a false economy to try do-it-yourself when it comes to vibrators or dildoes. It may seem preferable to use a rounded top of a deodorant bottle – just the right size, shape and texture. Or even a battery-driven toothbrush. The danger is that, being shorter than a vibrator and not having a firm handhold, you can lose it. If you are experimenting with anal sex, the "take care" is even stronger. Don't forget that the rectum is essentially one long tube, stretching from the anus to your mouth. You can lose something up it, as casualty officers in hospitals the world over can tell you.

LOVE EGGS

But vibrators and dildoes are not the only objects you can make use of to spark up your sex play. You could try Love Eggs, also called Geisha Balls. Love Eggs are two hollow balls joined by a cord. They can contain smaller balls or weights that shift and move around inside them. The idea is to put these into the vagina, where they are reputed to keep a woman in a prolonged state of sexual arousal or even bring her to a climax. The reason is that the network of nerves that surrounds the vagina is connected to the prime site of sexual pleasure in a woman – the clitoris. The subtle but continuous pressure and movement of the balls can indeed produce highly effective stimulation. It's suggested that women can slip them inside and then go about their ordinary business. Any movement makes the weights inside shift around, increasing sensation. Some women find Love Eggs give an amazing boost to their sex lives. You can use them on your own, to arouse and satisfy you in themselves, or to arouse you before pleasing yourself through masturbation. Or you can use them as foreplay, before making love with your partner. It has to be said, however, that some women say they do nothing for sexual sensation and feel irritating, as if the wearer was permanently on the verge of losing a tampon.

A cheap, easy and very effective and enjoyable sex toy is a feather. You can use a single feather, and try tracing the veins on your partner's body, up and down their arms and legs, inside elbows and the backs of knees, across the neck and top of the shoulders, around nipples and genitals. Or you could use a bunch of soft feathers and tickle his penis or her clitoris, or nipples on both of you. Stop there, however. It's been said that using a feather to arouse your partner is a perfect definition of erotic. The definition of kinky is when you use the whole chicken!

TURN YOUR BACK

Many people find anal stimulation intensely exciting. This is why using a vibrator around the back passage can be pleasurable. There are, however, several types of sex toy that capitalize on this. Thai beads and butt plugs are two. Thai beads are the anal version of Love Eggs and can be used by men or women who find the anal area sensitive and that stimulating it is sexually arousing. Thai beads are a series of plastic, metal or wooden beads on a string, plastic thread or flexible rod. The idea is to insert this into the rectum and move them in and out or vibrate them by gently flicking the rod. As you climax, you slowly or suddenly pull them out, which intensifies the sensations.

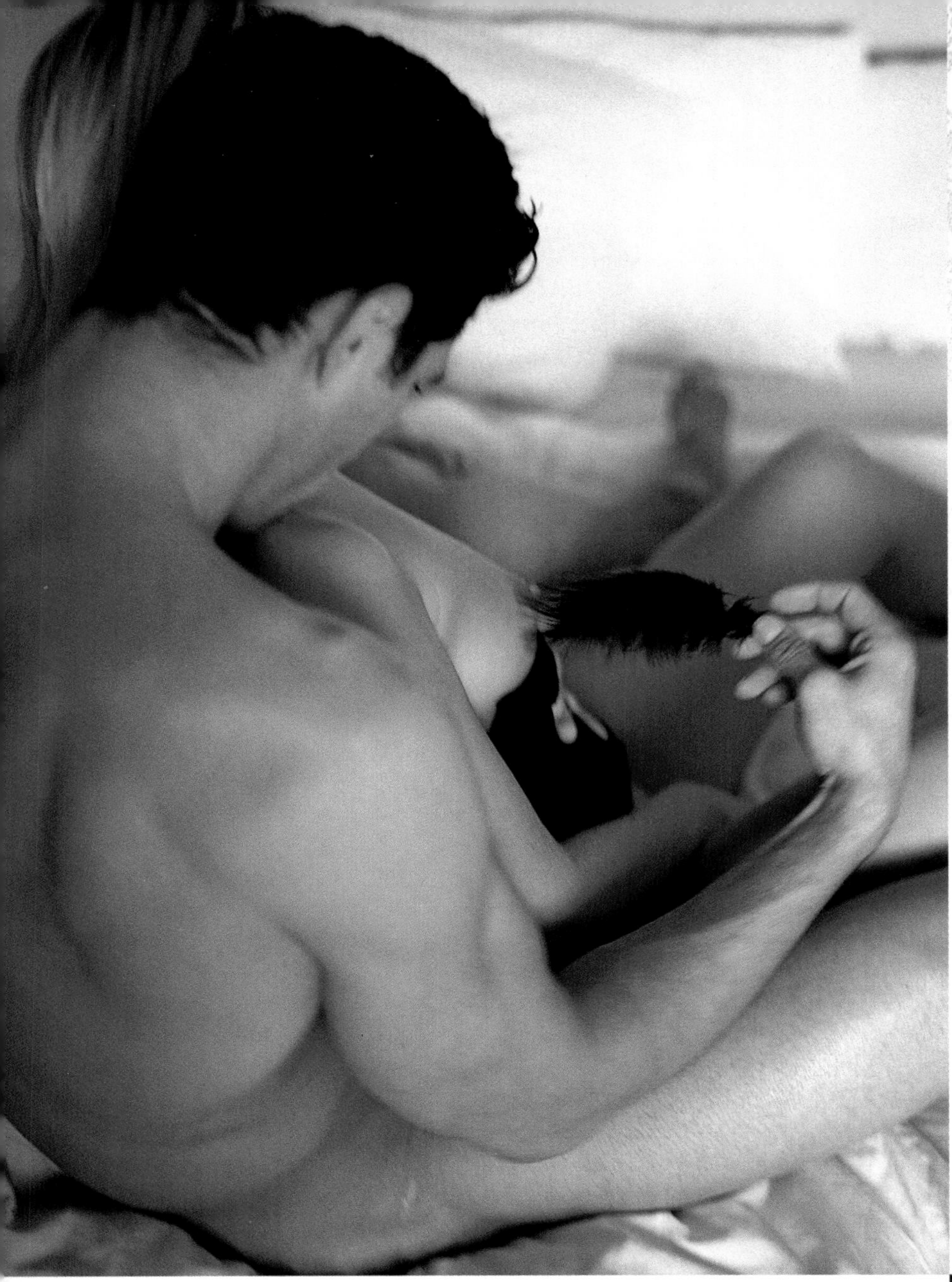

You can use a single feather, and try tracing the veins on your partner's body, up and down their arms and legs, inside elbows and the backs of knees, across the neck and top of the shoulders, around nipples and genitals.

A cheap, easy and very effective and enjoyable sex toy is a feather.

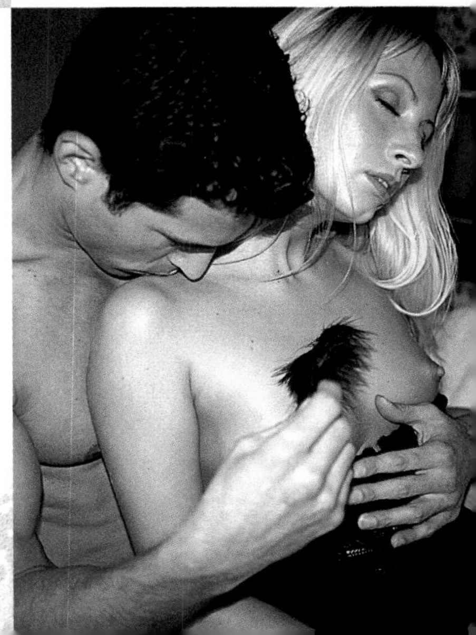

Another anal stimulator is the butt plug. Butt plugs are like vibrators, but are thicker and shorter. They have a widened end plate or a longer handgrip, to make sure you don't lose them. Unlike the vagina, the back passage extends far inside the body. It is possible to lose something inside you if you insert it too far – as generations of casualty doctors and nurses can tell you! ("Slipped and fell over in the kitchen and just happened to fall on the sauce bottle. Of course you did, sir. Funny it's got a condom on it.")

A HELPING HAND

Sex toys and aids can also come to your rescue if the spirit is willing but the flesh weak. If his body is letting him down at the vital moment, or if the couple would like to give nature a hand in either promoting or maintaining an erection, Arab straps and penis rings can do so. When a man has an erection, blood rushes into the area, filling special spongy tissue in his penis, swelling and stiffening it. When he climaxes, the blood drains away and the tissue becomes soft once again. Problems arise if the blood drains away too quickly and the penis never fully becomes hard or he becomes soft too early for either of their tastes. If you put something tight around the base of the penis during or after an erection, you can prevent the blood from draining away and so keep the erection harder for longer. Arab straps, penis or so-called "cock-and-ball" rings all do the same, strengthening and maintaining a man's erection. These are devices made of leather, metal and/or rubber. The idea is to stimulate the man so he becomes hard and then can fasten a strap or series of straps or slip over a flexible ring so it grips around the base of the penis. Arab straps and cock-and-ball rings also grip around the shaft of the penis and the scrotum.

If you need some help to get an erection, another useful sex aid is the male developer. They work on the vacuum principle. The idea is to insert the penis into a plastic cylinder which has a rubber seal that fits snugly around the base of the penis, making the tube airtight. The other end of the cylinder has a tube that goes to a manual or electric pump. As

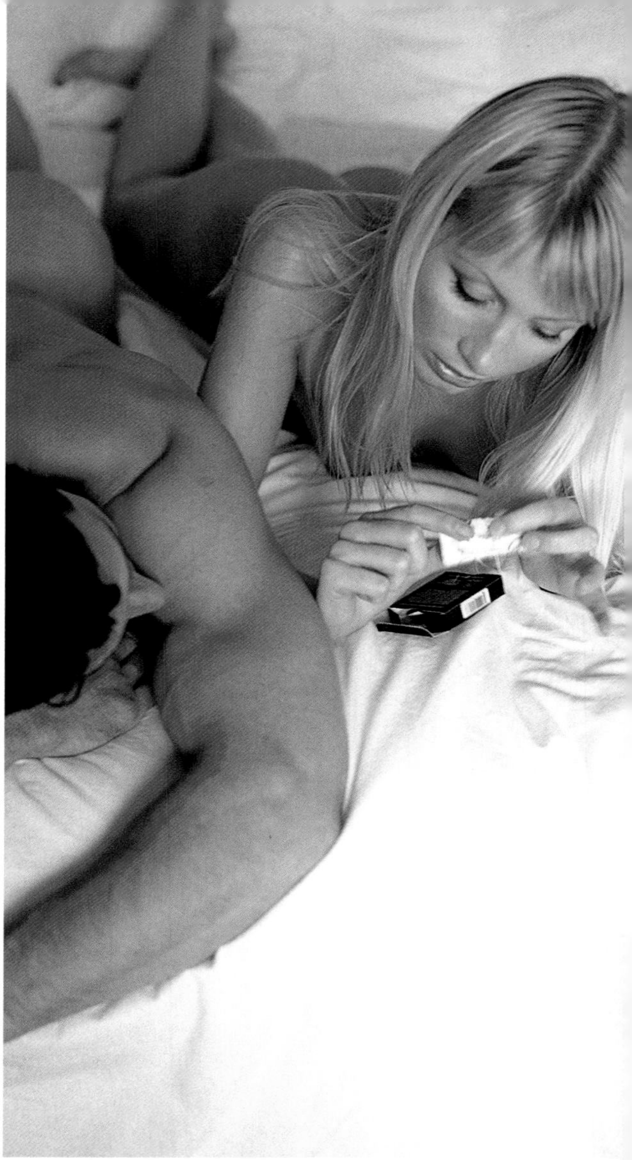

A helping hand when only the spirit is willing

There is quite a range of products to add sensation for the partner who is being penetrated. Penis sleeves, condoms with bumps and ribs and rings.

you pump air out, creating a vacuum, blood is drawn into the penis and, bingo, you have a hard-on that's meant to be, and often is, bigger and harder than usual. The sellers of vacuum pumps usually promise that they will enlarge the penis, and imply this means for keeps. This sounds very promising, but whatever they say the effect is only temporary. Unless you use a ring or strap to keep that blood in, poor little John Thomas goes back to his usual size when you take the developer off. And no matter how often you pump him up in this way, he's not going to get any bigger for good. But the technique is invaluable if the man is having difficulties in getting or maintaining an erection and by using this in conjunction with a strap or ring can certainly make a difference to your lovemaking.

EXTRA SENSATION

There is quite a range of products to add sensation for the partner who is being penetrated. Penis sleeves, condoms with bumps and ribs, rings that fit all the way down the shaft and rest at the base of the penis can all be used to increase sensation inside the vagina or anus and on the clitoris. "The Gates of Hell", for instance, are a number of rings that can be slipped along the shaft of the penis and will rub against the side of the sex or back passage as the couple make love. And women often find that Arab straps provide clitoral stimulation as the couple move together. Clit rings are also helpful in providing clitoral stimulation. These are tight, latex straps which fit around the base of the penis. They hold a pad or spiky protuberance against his body that rubs against the woman's clitoris. They can look pretty fearsome but many women find them highly enjoyable. Another condom variation is penile extensions. These have padded tips or are padded and re-enforced all over to add length and width to a man's pride and joy. The all-over sheath can, of course, be helpful when the couple want to go on making love after he has softened and would rather they could feel it was the man who was satisfying her rather than a vibrator. You can also improve on Nature with finger sleeves. These are short, rubber toys covered in bumps and lumps that you slip over his or her fingers and use to stimulate her clitoris or either of their back passages. If you are going to give these a try remember not to touch any other genital area after you have been stimulating the back passage.

If you might have been interested in the stimulation offered by genital or nipple piercings but are not keen on going the whole hog and having either pierced for your sexual pleasure, there are sex toys to give you temporary sensations in this way. There are clamps that you can attach to many different parts of the body. These come with chains attached which you can gently tug and vibrate to give the desired effect.

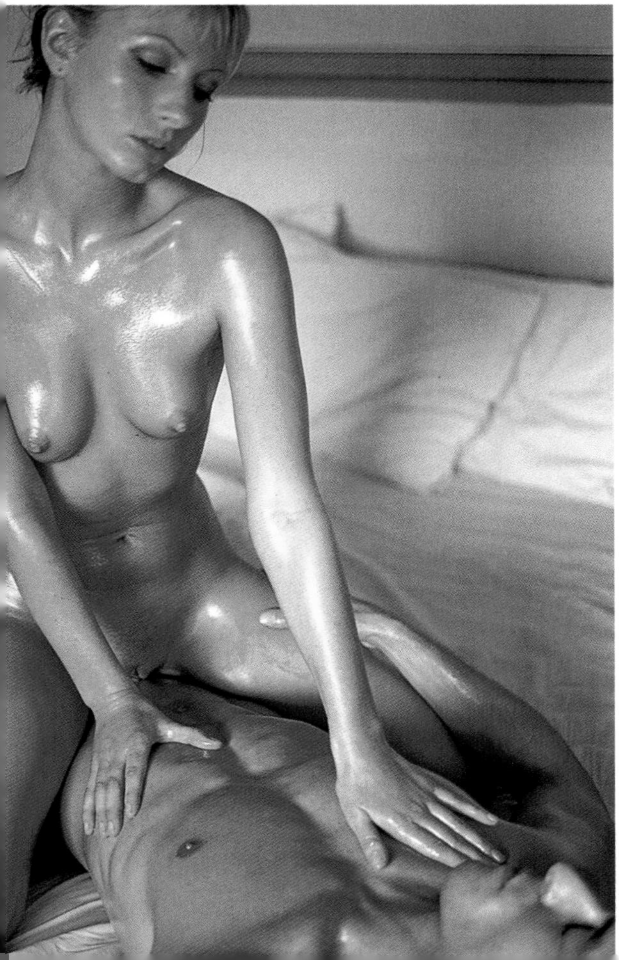

LOTIONS AND POTIONS

If you are looking for other toys to pep up your sex lives you may also want to stray into the field of creams, sprays and oils. Most sex toy outlets offer heat creams and sprays that are said to make you feel warm and itching to go. Lotions and potions that are meant to excite the sexual interest are hardly new. Roman enthusiasts recommended bathing the genitals in nasturtium juice and then

Left: Smooth your way to love with lotions and potions

beating them gently with nettles! The modern equivalents are a bit less painful. These contain chemicals that slightly inflame or irritate the skin surface and you rub them in or spray them on and wait for the results. The heat ingredient is actually the same stuff you would find in those pain-relieving balms in the sports medicine section of your pharmacy, although these use three to four times the amount of the active ingredient as those sold in sex shops. So if you were tempted to do-it-yourself, dilute with handcream and go carefully.

Heat creams and sprays are supposed to pep you up and speed you along, while the other forms of lotion or potion – the so-called "stud" creams – are meant to slow you down. The creams contain a small amount of surface anaesthetic. They dull sensations and so are meant to allow a man to last longer. The disadvantage is that the man can't feel much until the effects wear off and making love with a frozen penis rather defeats the object of the exercise. It can also be too much of a good thing. If he grinds on for several hours, his partner can be reduced to looking at the cracks in the ceiling or the stains on the carpet and the result can be friction burns rather than ecstatic enjoyment. It can be very useful, however, for men who have a problem with a quick-off-the-mark climax. If your early experience of sex was hurried and furtive, with pressure to get it over quickly in case you were interrupted, you will have been trained to be a premature ejaculator. Nervousness and performance anxiety early on in a relationship can have the same effect. Once you've had a few miss-hits the fear of failing again in the same way and the anticipation of a too-quick climax can make it a self-fulfilling prophecy. Breaking the cycle a few times can help a man last longer without the need for the cream.

There are two warnings here. One is that it may take ten to fifteen minutes for the anaesthetic to have some effect, so it's a good idea to spray on or rub in at the beginning of love play and then wait a while before having penetrative sex. Enjoy yourself for a delicious preliminary time before getting it together. It's also important not to pass the substance on the penis to the vagina or clitoris – he's the one who wants to go slow, not her. Women tend not to have a problem with premature ejaculation since if they climax as soon as sex starts, they can simply go on to have another...and another. So it's a good idea to use a condom over the frozen member. It's also worth noting that the ingredient in stud creams is exactly the same as that found in minor wound, teething or sore mouth remedies. If you want to save money or blushes when buying it, try one of those. It's not quite the same as anointing yourself with something from a jar, tub or tube marked "Rampant Sexy Animal" but it's a hell of a lot cheaper.

Doctors and Nurses can be an excellent game for big boys and girls, too. It allows you the perfect opportunity to twiddle this and tweak that, to stroke and knead with impunity.

Lubrication creams and oils can also add a lot to your lovemaking: when they are smoothed on the body they encourage sensual massage. But they can also be useful when extra lubrication is needed for penetrative sex, whether vaginal or anal. It's just important to note that any oil or oil-based cream or jelly will destroy the rubber or latex of any barrier method of contraception at a frightening rate. The female condom, being made of polyurethane, is safe. But most condoms and diaphragms will quite literally dissolve before your very eyes in a matter of minutes. So if you are using one for safer sex, against infection or

Right: Dressing up and using fantasy can give a sparkle to a couple's sex games

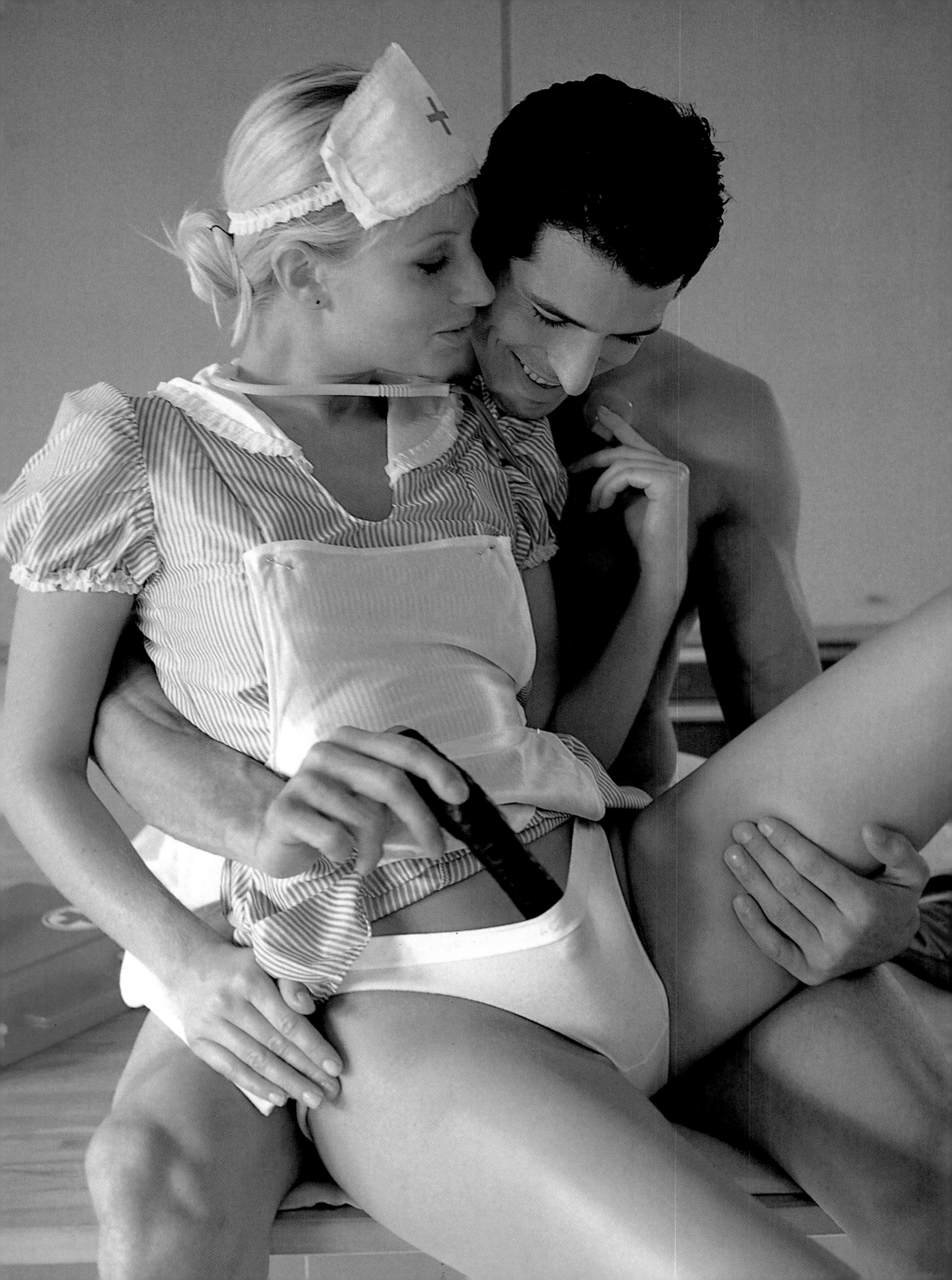

pregnancy, be sure to use a water-based lubricating product from the pharmacist which is designed to be used in lovemaking.

If you'd like to experiment with some sex toys, try a fantasy game to get you started. Having the confidence to use them can take some effort. Most of us suffer from the sneaking feeling that enjoying sex is not allowed. Our first, early, explorations of our bodies were probably met with slapped hands and a telling off. We knew that authority, in the form of our parents, didn't approve. Children often get round the prohibitions on sex play with the very popular game of Doctors and Nurses. It's such a good excuse to let those hands roam free, as they find out what feels good and which parts of the body differ from little girls to little boys. Most young people play Doctors and Nurses at some time, as a cover for early sexual curiosity. We know that medical personnel are only doing their job when they have you on the couch, undressed, and open to their examination. If you were a doctor or a nurse, it would be perfectly OK for you to have your hands all over the unclothed body of your patient. It's also OK for a patient to be seen by a doctor, even when they may feel too shy to be seen by anyone else. Doctors and Nurses can be an excellent game for big boys and girls, too. It allows you the perfect opportunity to twiddle this and tweak that, to stroke and knead with impunity. After all, doctor is only doing his or her job, examining the patient to make it all better. And the patient is only doing the proper thing in turn, by lying there and accepting doctor's administrations, and helping out by indicating where it hurts and where it does not. But there is a special reason why Doctors and Nurses is such a good way of letting you start some discoveries with sex toys. As far back as the first century, the Greek physician Galen came up with the wonderful idea (for him or for her we will never know) that rubbing a woman's vulva was a sure-fire cure for her hysteria. Hysteria and women were synonymous in early times and both Hippocrates and Plato subscribed to this view. They saw marriage as the only real answer and cure for hysteria but also thought that vulvic massage ran it a pretty close second. Not surprisingly, male doctors of the time claimed this massage was a difficult technique to learn. They claimed it needed constant practice and frequent rehearsal. You can imagine the scene with the wide-eyed doctor saying to his equally ecstatic patient, for the third time that session, "Just lie back once more, Mrs Papadopulos, and we'll see if we can try that again, shall we?"

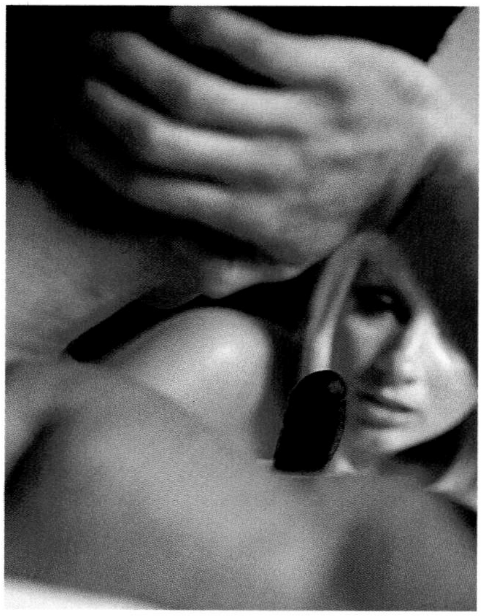
Just follow doctor's orders

Set the scene by arranging your chosen room as an examination cubicle. Have a single divan, sofa or table covered with a towel or sheet, to stand in for the examination couch. Lay out a tray of instruments – a container of lubricating cream, jelly or oil, surgical gloves, a vibrator. You can really make that hospital atmosphere come alive with a visit to your pharmacy. Buy some surgical gloves and snap them on, not forgetting to wash your hands thoroughly beforehand to get in the mood – very ER! And get some hospital disinfectant to splash on the towel or sheet for a really authentic smell that will transport you to your local A&E. Get your uniforms prepared. You're to be doctor and nurse in a busy hospital. Don't forget that there are male nurses and female doctors, so you can try this taking your turns in either role. One of you is in a doctor's white jacket, or in the "scrubs" worn for operating theatre; green or blue loose cotton jacket and tie-waist trousers. The other in a plain shirt and skirt/trousers for nurses uniform or could also be in "scrubs". Doctor is the one in authority, someone nurse admires and will listen to. Anything a doctor suggests must be for your own good, so the nurse is going to pay heed and follow the doctor's suggestions.

Anything a doctor suggests must be for your own good, so the nurse is going to pay heed and follow the doctor's suggestions.

Start the action by imagining it's been a hard night. As nurse passes the doctor's room, the doctor calls out, "You look worn out, nurse. Got a headache?" "Yes, doctor, I can't seem to get rid of it." "Well, I know a cure for that, nurse. Hop up on the couch and I'll give you a neck massage." Nurse lies down and the doctor says, "I'm really good at relieving tension this way, nurse, just tell me if this feels good." Doctor then proceeds to stroke and massage nurse's neck and back, unbuttoning and pushing down or pulling up nurse's uniform to reach. Grateful nurse can say, "Oh, doctor, you do have healing hands." To keep in role, both of you should only address each other as "doctor" and "nurse". As doctor strokes nurse's neck and back, one hand strays to other parts of the body. "You're really tense, nurse, you should have a proper massage, you know. I read in an old medical book that this can help." It's actually true that the Victorians believed that tension resulted from what they called congestion. Congestion, they thought, was relieved when the sexual organs were massaged to the point where the patient became suddenly relaxed and relieved. So doctor should produce a vibrator, and after gently unbuttoning nurse's uniform, proceed to give medically prescribed treatment. Doctor can press the buzzing vibrator to nurse's nipples, down the belly and around the genitals, asking, "Does this feel better ?" Nurse can say, "Oh yes, doctor. But it really does feel tense here…and here…and here," showing doctor where it hurts and where best to give help. Doctor can use a feather in the absence of a vibrator, or both.

Playing this sort of fantasy game to allow you to experiment certainly works for many couples. Kofi and Efia had a happy and loving sex life, but Efia would never let her partner see her naked. She had come away from her childhood feeling shy about herself and convinced that she was ugly and too fat. She was terrified of letting Kofi see her without clothes in case he wasn't attracted to her. And she was scared of "letting go" and really enjoying herself in sex, thinking it would somehow be wrong. She could remember playing Doctors and Nurses as a child – and the almighty telling off it earned her! So Kofi's suggestion they try it at first made her recoil. And then she realized it also made her feel quite excited. It would be like re-running her past, by going back and doing something she remembered with shame but could now feel was OK. When they re-enacted the scene, she found she was able to take her clothes off in full light, and didn't mind having Kofi see her. She could not only let "Doctor Kofi" do a full examination, but also arouse her. Under doctor's orders, Efia was able to relax and allow herself to respond.

IT'S NO LAUGHING MATTER

It's a great pity that sex toys are still considered by some people to be either a bit of a joke or rather sleazy. Many of the catalogues produced by commercial firms don't help here, being lurid, sexist, tacky and trashy. Some of the shops can be seen by people who would like to buy as being places where they would feel uncomfortable to go. What could and should be fun becomes furtive, so embarrassment often holds people back from getting the things they would love to share together. Fortunately there has been quite a sea change in the last year or so. America started this by offering both shops and mail-order services by women and for women, with smart, well-designed catalogues that were far removed from the almost pornographic conventional kind. Sex toys are now not only available on the Internet but there are also excellent companies in the UK – one company has also done a lot to make sex toy shopping a fun affair by selling mainly through parties. And now the ultra-respectable charity the Family Planning Association, recognizing the role of sex toys in many people's lives, is offering guaranteed products through its own mail-order company. There's never been a better time to find out if they could do something for your sex life.

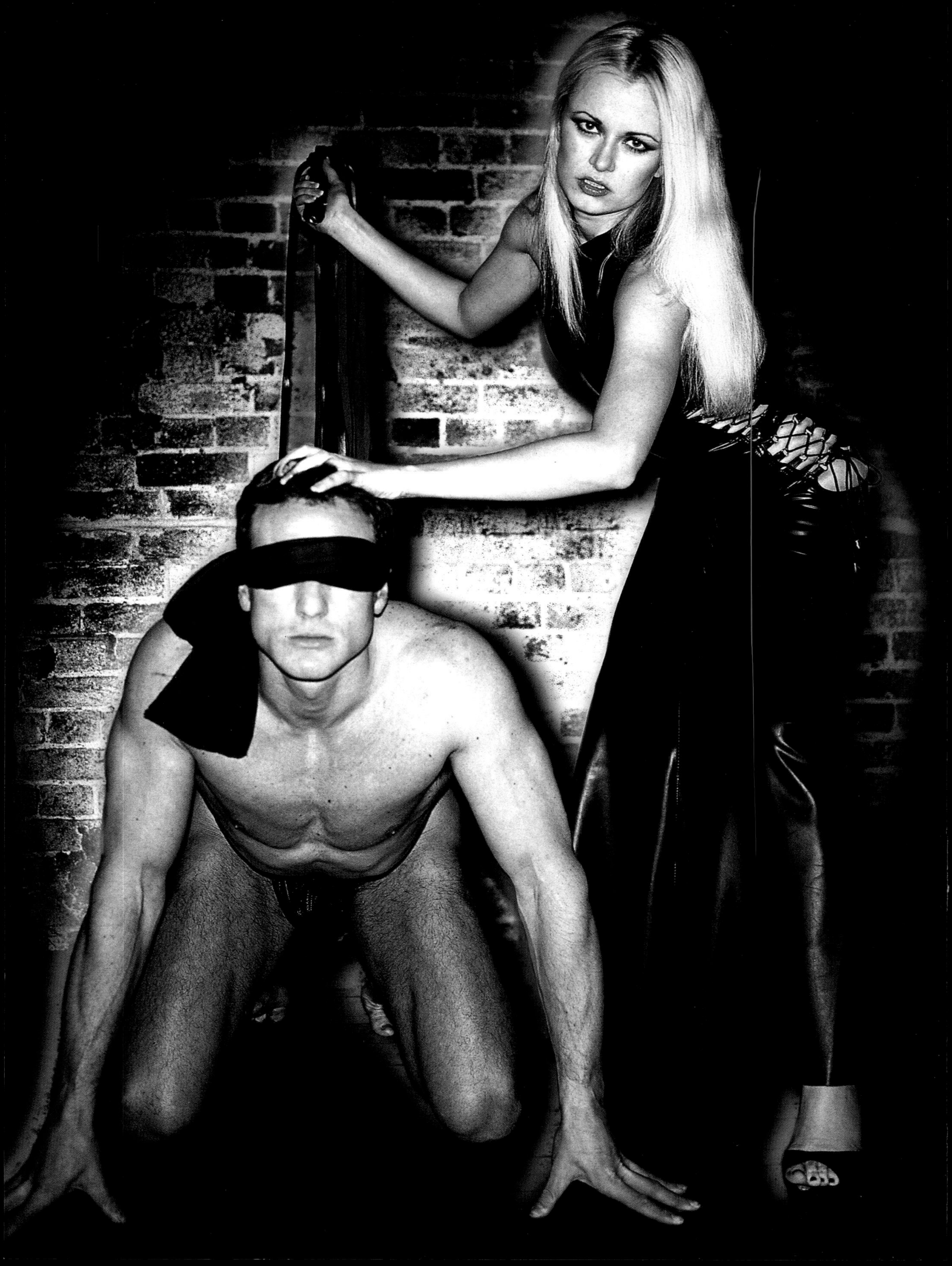

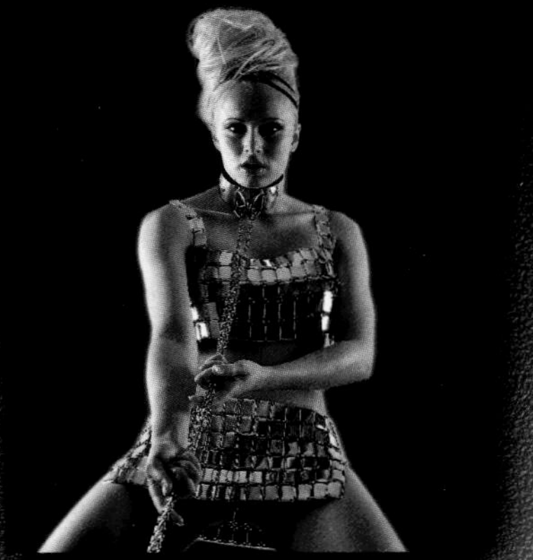

Chapter 5

DOMINATE ME

So, you've set the scene for sex and explored both dressing and undressing, and maybe even incorporating sex toys into your sexual repertoire. What would be the next step to unleashing your hidden, adventurous side? Strange as it may sound, one way of really letting you and your partner loose and unlocking your imaginations may be to experiment with tying each other up.

The world of bondage, sub/doms, S&M and B&D is said by many to be the ultimate way of allowing sexual repression to be left behind and true sexual innovation and enjoyment to come out. Bondage is a sexual variation or game in which restraints such as ropes, chains, cloth or leather straps are used to bind, tie or hold a sexual partner.

When you're using mild bondage to enliven a sexual fantasy it's often called restraint rather than bondage. The person doing the binding is considered "dominant" while the person being bound is considered "submissive" and this sexual variation is also known as sub/dom. Sub/dom sexual relationships are those in which one partner assumes total control and the other does exactly as they are told. If you're dabbling in this field, you may also hear the terms B&D or Master/Slave. The

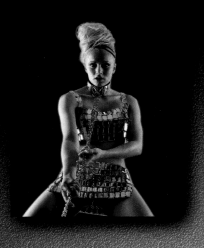

"D" stands for discipline, in which one partner not only dominates the other – a willing participant – but dishes out physical punishment to the submissive partner. The chastisement can range from physical restraint to mild spankings to painful beatings. This is usually administered with a cane made of bamboo or other light wood, a whip or a paddle. Getting a kick out of giving or receiving pain and humiliation is known as S&M – sado-masochism – where the submissive partner gets their kicks from having pain inflicted and the dominant one gets theirs from dishing out the punishment. Or, as the old joke goes "The masochist says 'Beat me!' and the sadist says 'No!'". But sub/dom can be totally painless, with humiliation being the point of the exercise rather than crude physical stuff. Taken to an extreme, bondage sex fringes over into the fetish scene. Fetish sex is when someone is sexually aroused and takes sexual pleasure through use of something or some activity or a part of the body that isn't usually seen as suggestive. Fetish objects may be shoes or cigarette lighters; a fetish action may be brushing your hair; and someone with a fetish may be turned on by your toes or fingers rather than your breasts or penis. When the leather clothes or the whip or the bullying act arouses you, far more than your partner themselves or any sex act between you, you're leaning over into fetish sex.

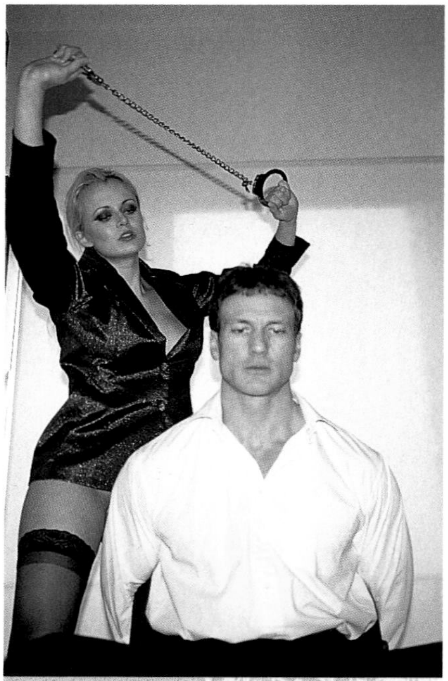

There's a bit of submissive/ dominant in most people.

BE UNKIND TO ME

There's a bit of the sub/dom in most people. How often have you got a kick out of telling those around you what to do? And isn't it relaxing, sometimes, to know someone else is taking total responsibility and running the show? When it comes to sex, you might be surprised to discover exactly how far you could take both impulses. You'll never know how much it could appeal to you unless you try. You can try out sub/dom carefully at first. Next time you make love, have one of you take the lead – and by that, I mean totally. The one to take the initiative, the dom, should make the advance, hustle their partner into sex, direct the action and be the one choosing what you do, where, when and for how long. If one of you is usually the one who makes the first move, let it be the other who tries this out. The dom needs to make a conscious effort to be arrogant, dictating and imperious. There are no "please" or "thank you" in sub/dom sex play. The idea is for the leader to demand exactly what they want, and to mete out appropriate punishment if they don't get it. Doms are not, however, unreasonable. If the slave performs well, he or she will be allowed to have their own pleasure too. You could also experiment with verbal rather than physical domineering. Plenty of couples like each other to "talk dirty" when they make love. Asking

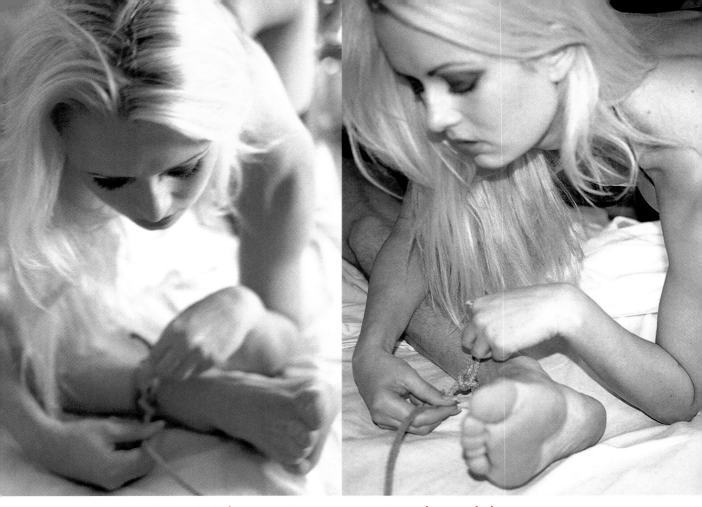

Once you're tied up, you can't say no as your partner explores your body

for or describing what you'd like to do to each other, in the most basic of terms, can get those juices flowing. But some people also find it arousing to talk dirty in another way, not only to use obscenities but also put-downs and hurtful or embarrassing secrets. You could start with mild criticism and if both of you feel comfortable, work up to total, if ritual, humiliation, telling the other one off in a way that makes them feel really small. It can be sexually exciting because the one being told off can feel cleansed, as if they've had their punishment, paid the price and can now indulge in naughty thoughts and acts, since they now have permission to enjoy sex.

If you find a small taster of sub/dom sex play feels good, next time go a step further. Take the lead again, but this time use a scarf or belt and twist it round your partner's wrists, holding them down with their arms above their head and unable to use their hands as you have sex. If so far, so good, go even further afterward and the next time you have sex, tie your partner up. This time, use a scarf or belt or even some rope or cord. You could lash their hands behind their back or above their head. Or, you could tie them spread-eagled on the bed, to bedposts if you have them, to the legs of the bed by long cords if not. Take it in turns to be the one dominating. Think about, and talk over, how it feels. Do you find it scary to be in either position, and is it a fear that makes you want to stop, or one that drives you on? Does either situation give you a kick? Is sex better in either role?

PUNISH ME

Submissive and dominant sex play carries particular appeal for many people for special reasons to do with the way we often learn about sex. Many of us have our early sexual experiences spoiled by punishment and disapproval. When, as babies, we delighted in discovering our own bodies and the joys to be had from touching them, we often had our hands slapped. This can result in our feeling guilty, shy and embarrassed about our sexual desires or about our bodies. It means that people often find it difficult to relax into and allow their own sexual desires. Playing the submissive in a sex game is a way of ducking out from under those guilty feelings. If your master or mistress is telling you that you have to do it, if you are being threatened with punishments if you refuse and if you're tied up so you simply can't avoid what is happening to you, then you have no reason to feel guilty. What is happening to your body and how your body is responding is totally beyond your control. Many people who have found sex difficult to enjoy and their own sensuality hard to accept may discover bondage games can give them a whole new perspective. Being submissive can also be a particular relief to people who have to be strong, commanding and authoritative in their everyday lives. Many men who have high-powered jobs and can never let up being in command greatly enjoy taking on the passive role in their off times.

The other side of the coin is to be the one in charge. Taking the entire responsibility for being fully in control can also be immensely empowering. Being the dominant one means allowing for no rejection or criticism, no embarrassment or disagreement and is another way of drowning out any guilt or second thoughts. If your partner is tempted to be shocked at the way, or the fact that, you want to make love, you can simply stifle their objections with a spank or a slap. It's also immensely satisfying in itself and especially appeals to those who are usually at other people's beck and call.

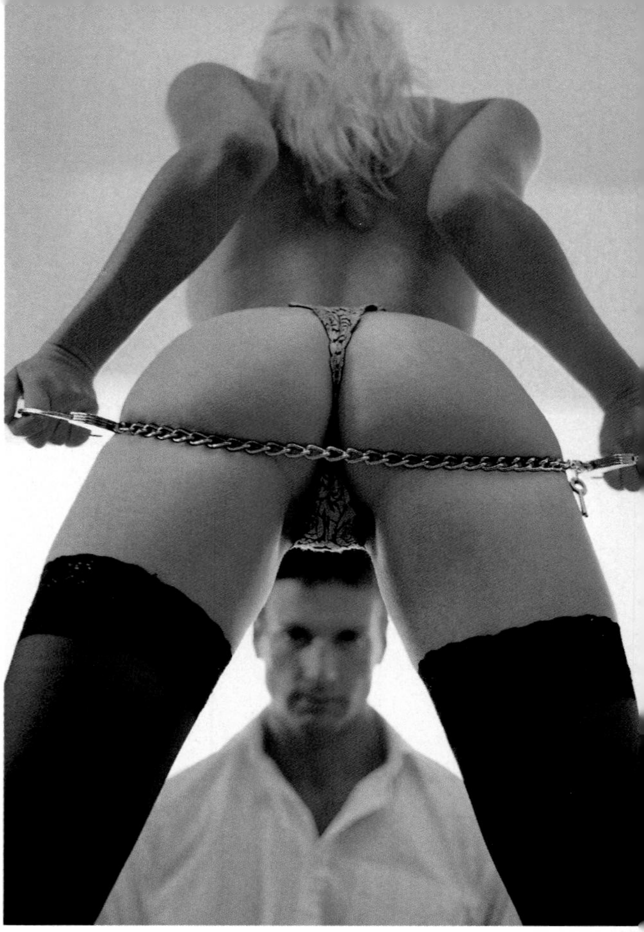

The joy of being told what to do

PLEASURE AND PAIN

There are several other reasons why pain inflicting games are so popular. Pleasure and pain are surprisingly close. When you become sexually aroused, your nipples, genitals and lips become engorged with blood, swell and heat up. When you

Many men who have high-powered jobs and can never let up being in command greatly enjoy taking on the passive role in their off times.

smack an arm, leg or buttock, it too smarts and becomes hot and sensitive. Make your buttocks tingle from a spanking, and your mind will often become confused, telling your body that the sensation is actually arousal. Plenty of people find it highly stirring to have small, measured and controlled amounts of pain inflicted during sex play by their partners. Another is that having pain inflicted upon you can be seen as a test. The "victims" vie to see how much they can bear, and how dangerous they can make the game and still survive. Coming through in once piece is felt to be an achievement, which lifts the spirits – among other things.

Just as you can confuse the body by substituting pain for pleasure and pleasure for pain, S&M, sub/dom sex play also harnesses the tendency for human beings to find anger and fear arousing. Arousal, as we have already discussed, causes distinct physical changes in the body. The pupils widen, the heart races, breath comes quickly and the body sweats. All these symptoms of sexual excitement are also present when we are frightened or enraged. Some people find that making love is a good way of making up after a row. If they then learn that the row can be an effective prelude to particularly passionate sex, a pattern may be set. Arguing, after all, can be a short cut to arousal, and a quicker and more guaranteed way of raising the emotions than trying to be lovey-dovey and romantic. You can become addicted to the heightened feelings and find yourself provoking rows just to enjoy the sex that follows.

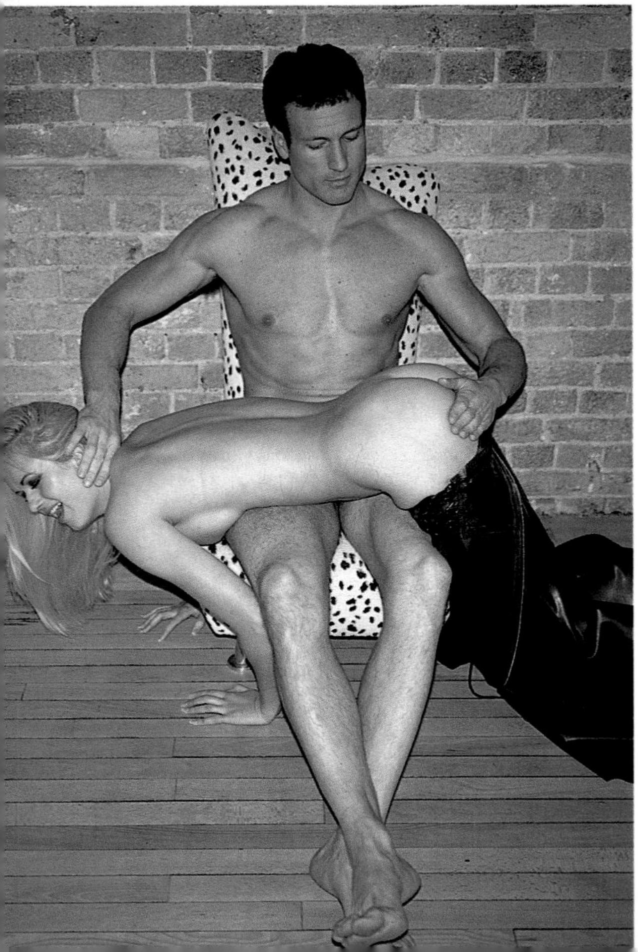

Make your buttocks tingle from a spanking, and your mind will often become confused, telling your body that the sensation is actually arousal.

BONDAGE AND FETISH SCENE

There is a huge variation in how far people are prepared to go in their sub/dom sex play and how much of the gear they will use or wear. The bondage and fetish scene tends to be associated with leather, rubber and latex. Over the last few years, of course, what once would have been considered very specialist gear has become almost High Street fashion. It started in the music scene, went through *haute couture* design and is now available in most department stores. After all, when leading department stores start commissioning bras, pants and suspenders from

Left: Pleasure and pain are very close

one of the leading sexy lingerie companies you know that it's moved from hard core into main stream. So what makes an outfit typically sub/dom? Think closely fitting, shiny textured and made from rubber, plastic, PVC, leather or latex. There should be straps, chains and as many metal studs as possible as well as zips and stiletto heels. The sound of the clothing is almost as important as the feel and it should creak, jingle and snap in a way that strikes fear or desire into the wearer and those around them. It should also smell of rubber, talc, sweat and other body fluids. If you are just a little bit into sub/dom, you may like the idea of leather boots, leather jeans, latex pants and maybe a studded collar or two. Go the whole hog and you or your partner will be kitted out from top to toe in form-fitting rubber, latex or PVC, or in a brief leather or rubber basque and suspenders or a studded leather harness and leather briefs, with nipple chains. Enthusiasts often take the bondage idea to interesting extremes, tying breasts or penises up with leather straps, cords or chains.

You can get a lot of the leather, latex or even rubber clothing from fashion or biker shops. If you want to get a little more specialist, then sex shops will obviously have most of the things you want and you can also find further contacts and manufacturers through the ads in "top shelf" magazines. Of course, the best source of all in these modern times is the Internet – just enter "bondage" or "fetish" and see what you find! You can also buy handcuffs or custom-made restraints to extend the fantasy. There are chains and padlocks, padded leather wrist and ankle cuffs and collars. You can have harnesses made of metal, rope and leather that tie hands behind the back or to the waist, thighs, ankles or neck. There are blindfolds and gags, and spreader bars that fasten to wrists, thighs and ankles to force and keep them apart. You can even buy harnesses, racks and scaffolds. If you want a taste of the more expensive equipment, you can even book into specialist hotels that offer "dungeons" for their guests' use.

MEET THE NEIGHBOURS

Enthusiasts often meet each other in clubs or at private parties where sub/dom behaviour can either just be hinted at as a way of attracting a partner for private games or where people strut their stuff in front of each other as a way of adding a kick to what goes on between the two of them. Some indulge in intense competition with each other by showing off their master/mistress or slave and exactly how far they will go to dominate or be dominated. In some places, for instance, couples will enter into whipping matches, comparing the artistry with which the dom disciplines their sub or simply, crudely comparing how much punishment they can take. Most fetish and sub/dom clubs are run under very strict conditions. There are rules covering all behaviour and regulars to the scene say that you are less likely to be hassled unpleasantly here than you could be in an ordinary bar. If you want to learn the rules and pick up some tips, you could do worse than visit one, watch and listen. Since the public sub/dom scene is a mixture of exhibitionism and voyeurism, your interest will not be resented as long as you aren't a tourist, only along to stare and laugh.

Ask your partner which parts they find attractive, and look at that part of your body with a new appreciation.

♦ TRY THIS

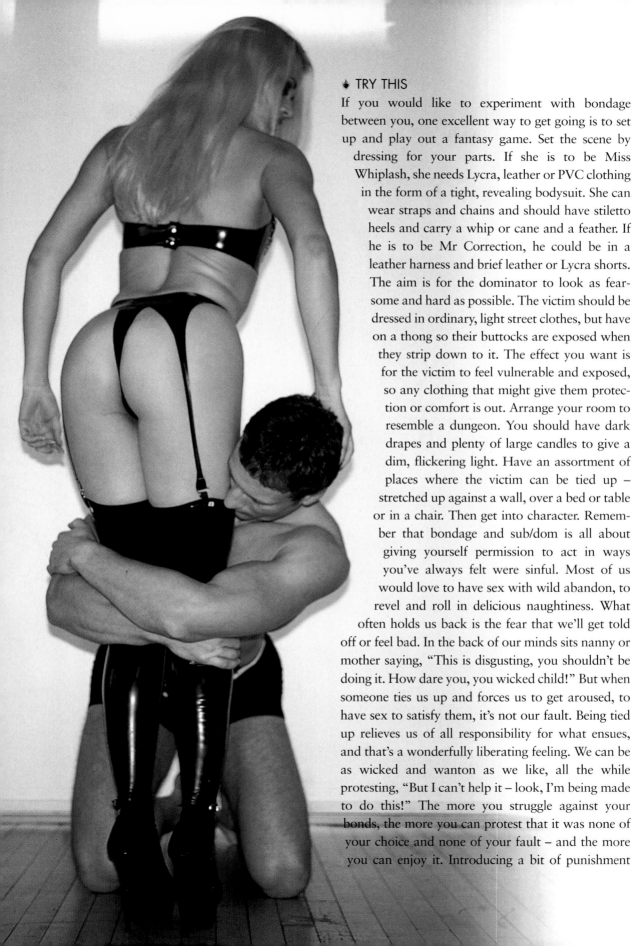

If you would like to experiment with bondage between you, one excellent way to get going is to set up and play out a fantasy game. Set the scene by dressing for your parts. If she is to be Miss Whiplash, she needs Lycra, leather or PVC clothing in the form of a tight, revealing bodysuit. She can wear straps and chains and should have stiletto heels and carry a whip or cane and a feather. If he is to be Mr Correction, he could be in a leather harness and brief leather or Lycra shorts. The aim is for the dominator to look as fearsome and hard as possible. The victim should be dressed in ordinary, light street clothes, but have on a thong so their buttocks are exposed when they strip down to it. The effect you want is for the victim to feel vulnerable and exposed, so any clothing that might give them protection or comfort is out. Arrange your room to resemble a dungeon. You should have dark drapes and plenty of large candles to give a dim, flickering light. Have an assortment of places where the victim can be tied up – stretched up against a wall, over a bed or table or in a chair. Then get into character. Remember that bondage and sub/dom is all about giving yourself permission to act in ways you've always felt were sinful. Most of us would love to have sex with wild abandon, to revel and roll in delicious naughtiness. What often holds us back is the fear that we'll get told off or feel bad. In the back of our minds sits nanny or mother saying, "This is disgusting, you shouldn't be doing it. How dare you, you wicked child!" But when someone ties us up and forces us to get aroused, to have sex to satisfy them, it's not our fault. Being tied up relieves us of all responsibility for what ensues, and that's a wonderfully liberating feeling. We can be as wicked and wanton as we like, all the while protesting, "But I can't help it – look, I'm being made to do this!" The more you struggle against your bonds, the more you can protest that it was none of your choice and none of your fault – and the more you can enjoy it. Introducing a bit of punishment

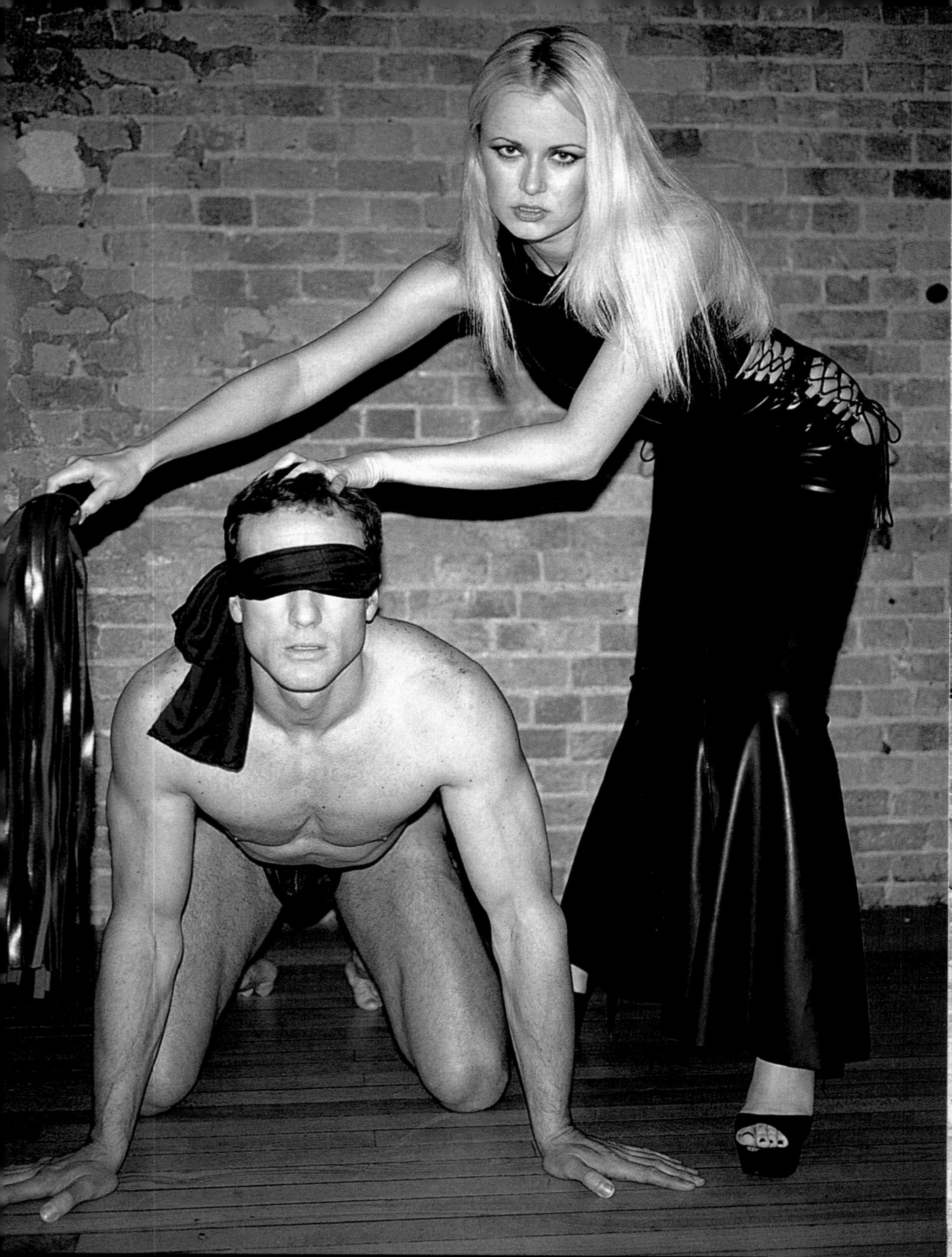

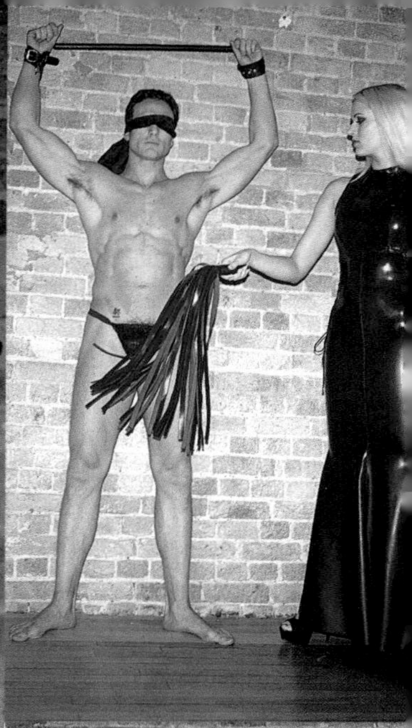

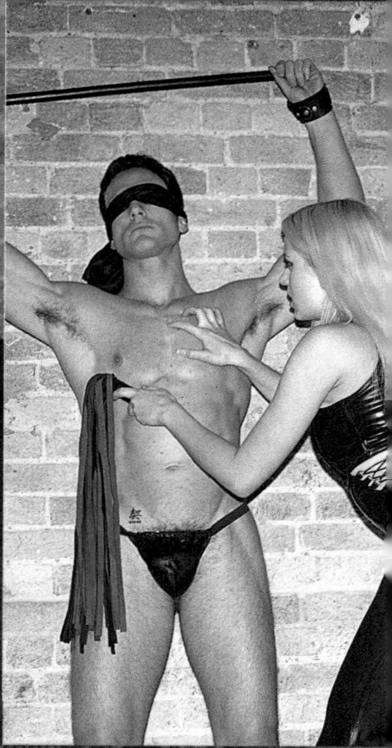

They've decided to pay a visit to Miss Whiplash/Mr Correction, and feel committed to this but are scared stiff of what they might find and what might happen.

into the game makes it even more comforting. As you are spanked or beaten, you can soothe any lingering feelings of guilt for enjoying what's happening. It's as if you say, "Yes, I know I'm being depraved, but look, I'm being punished so I don't have to feel bad about it." When you play this game, both of you are set free to enjoy yourselves with no misgivings or guilt. The victim is shivering with anticipation – scared yet excited. They've decided to pay a visit to Miss Whiplash/Mr Correction, and feel committed to this but are scared stiff of what they might find and what might happen. But the decision has been made and it's now out of their hands. The dominator has no fears and no concerns but is in charge – absolutely. They should be waiting, whip in hand and foot tapping.

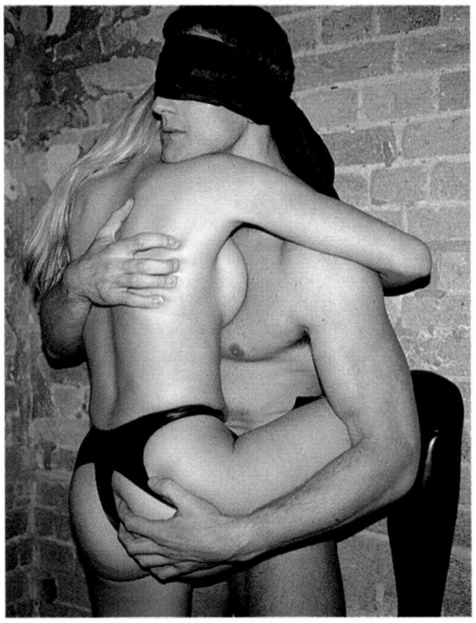

Helpless – and loving every moment

SPANKING FUN

Start the action by having the victim knock on the door, nervously. They are answered by a fearsome creature, who snaps, "Hello, worm. Come in, strip off, don't give me any lip and do as you're told." The dominator feels total certainty, is sure and in control. They know what the victim needs and are about to give it to them. The victim is led into the dungeon and made to strip down to a thong. As they take off each piece of clothing, the dominator prods the victim with the whip and sneers, "What a miserable body, you really do need some correction, don't you?" "Yes, Boss. Whatever you say, Boss." The victim is blindfolded and tied up and the dominator then uses either feather or whip, together or one after the other, to tickle and spank. "Don't get aroused or you'll be sorry," or "Don't you dare come without my permission," or "Come on, let's have a bit of action here," they'll demand as they arouse but delay the victim's climax. The dominator will take their own satisfaction from the victim's cringing body but the victim can only submit. They are allowed to come only when the dominator says they may.

Being relieved of responsibility by bondage sex play can help many couples. Ingrid and Tony found playing a sub/dom sex game transformed their marriage. Ingrid had been brought up to see sex as somehow dirty and perverse. She found it difficult to have an orgasm because whenever she found herself enjoying sex with Tony, she'd suddenly feel guilty and draw back. She had had orgasms while petting and, although she found it difficult to admit it, when exploring herself. But she had never actually come while having sex with Tony. They saw a sexual therapist and during one of their discussions, Ingrid hesitantly described a film scene she had once watched that had made her feel, as she put it, "funny, sort of jumpy inside". What she had felt was sexual arousal, and what she had seen was bondage. The next time they made love, Tony suddenly produced one of his ties and a belt and tied Ingrid to the bedstead. "I've got you helpless," he told her. "You can't stop me and nothing that now happens is up to you." Tony proceeded to tickle and suck Ingrid's nipples and to stroke her breasts and clitoris. Normally, when he tried to do this, Ingrid would enjoy and return his caresses up to a point and then suddenly

Left: Bondage games can set you free to enjoy yourselves

pull and turn away. This time, she could not. He slowly entered her, all the while flicking his tongue and fingers over her body, and telling her that he had her in his power and she had to do what she was told. By being tied up, Ingrid was released from feeling responsible for her enjoyment. By telling herself it wasn't her choice or her fault, she didn't have to feel guilty for the pleasure she was having from what Tony was doing. Ingrid had the first orgasm she had ever enjoyed during sex... and then her second, and third.

TAKING CARE

If you are going to use bondage as a part of your sexual repertoire, there are a few warnings you should pay heed to. Agree your limits in advance. Never be pushed into doing something you genuinely don't want to try. And never force your partner to do something that makes them uncomfortable. It is play, not reality, and this is something that can only be enjoyed by truly consenting adults. Anything else and it becomes abuse and sexual bullying. It's also absolutely vital that you have a code word to tell your partner that they or the game is getting beyond the bounds. Obviously, you want to be able to cry a pretend, "No, no, stop, let me go!" as part of the scenario, and have this plea ignored. But you also want to be able to say, "Now, I really mean it, let me go." The trick is to have an agreed word or phrase that you wouldn't ordinarily use – such as "rabbits" or "cold potatoes" to mean "LET ME OUT OF THIS, AT ONCE". And both of you have to promise, and keep to that promise, to pay attention and be trustworthy. Being tied tightly and even round the neck might be part of your scenario, but take care that the constraint isn't so tight that it really hurts or leaves marks. Gags may also be part of your agreed trappings, but use them with care. Whatever you use, never, ever constrict breathing. And make sure you can get out of the bonds. One urban myth about bondage is of the couple who handcuffed themselves, planning to spend the weekend trapped together. They sent the handcuff keys off in a self-addressed envelope, to arrive by Monday morning's post, in time to release themselves for work. Sadly, they didn't realize there was a postal strike, which lasted the entire week.

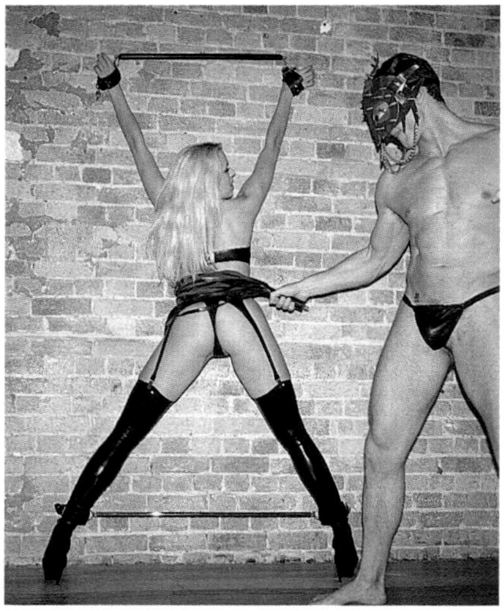

Agree your limits in advance and then relax

The trick is to have an agreed word or phrase that you wouldn't ordinarily use – such as "rabbits" or "cold potatoes" to mean "Let me out of this, at once".

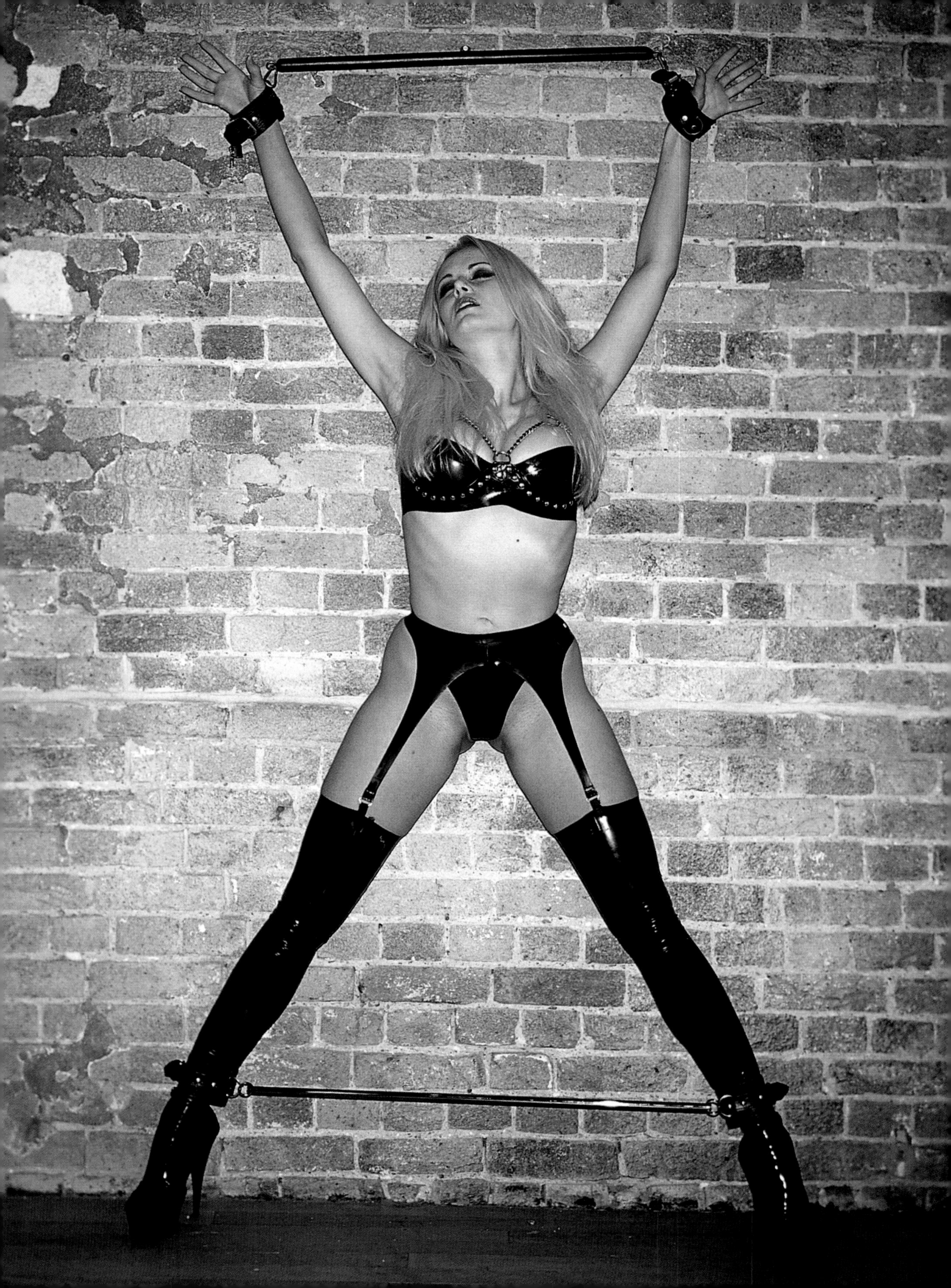

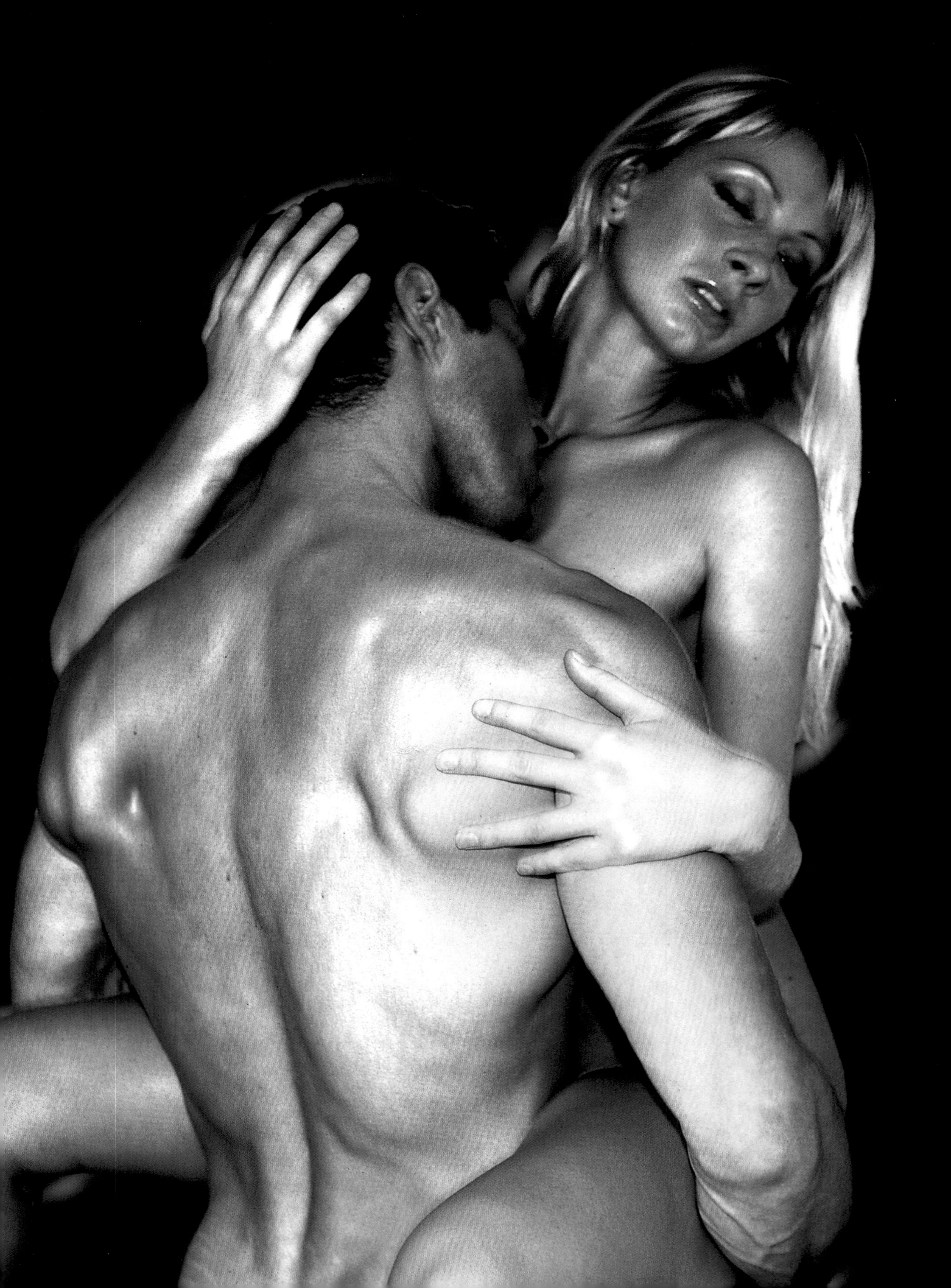

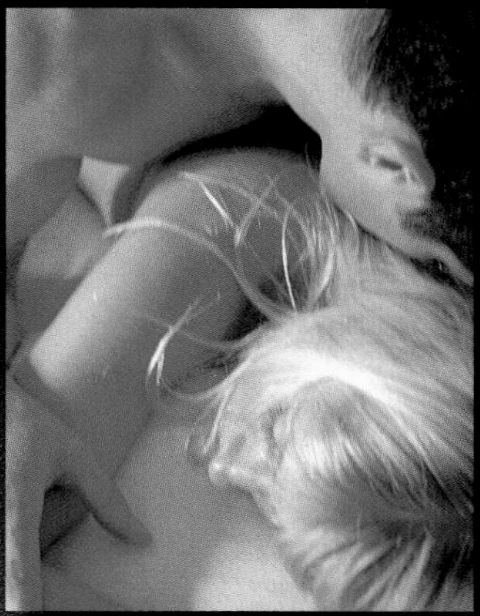

Chapter 6

POSITIONS OF THE NIGHT

There are many ways of making love. You can enjoy sex lying face-to-face with him on top and her below. If the two of you are concentrating on each other's needs and pleasures this can be exciting and satisfying. Some people call this "vanilla" or "meat and potatoes" sex and there's nothing wrong with that. But sometimes we prefer pistachio or double chocolate with sprinkles or we have a definite craving for caviar and champagne.

Different sexual positions can add flavour and savour to your sex life and bring a totally new dimension to your sexual adventures in several ways. One is that any change has you re-evaluating and rediscovering and thus enjoying a familiar experience as if it were new. When you are not going through well-tried and well-rehearsed motions you find yourself making all sorts of interesting findings. When you are trying out something new it requires you to ask questions and to give answers – to communicate, in other words. And communication is the fast track to better sex in your relationship. But there is yet another reason and this is that while you might think that one way of putting two bodies together would be the same as any other way, in fact different sexual positions can

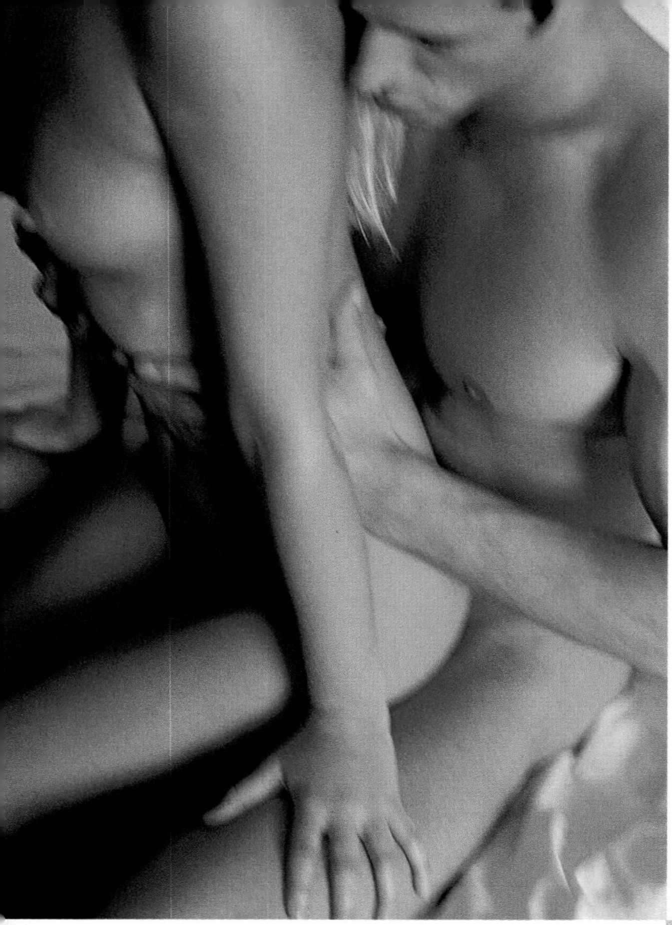

Above and right: Hands free to love and caress

500 SEXUAL POSITIONS

Different sexual positions have been written about by commentators for at least two thousand years, but our fascination goes back much further than that. Prehistoric cave paintings have been discovered that seem to depict a range of different positions for intercourse. Perhaps the most famous texts most of us know about are the *Kama Sutra*, written sometime between fifteen to nineteen hundred years ago in Hindi, and *The Perfumed Garden*, an Arabic treatise that is about a thousand years old. The *Kama Sutra* suggested eight basic love-making positions, while *The Perfumed Garden* said there were eleven. By putting them and many other texts together, certain researchers suggest that there are well over five hundred positions, each a slight variation on the other. Working your way through them all you are certainly unlikely to get bored, with enough to keep you going for at least a year without any repetition. Positions range from the athletic to the downright exotic.

open up new sensations. Some sexual positions give us a thrill because of our attitude toward them – they seem to be rather naughty and thus more exciting. Some, however, actually afford increased sexual sensation to men and women or both. The only thing that may hold you back from trying out something new is shyness, embarrassment or lack of self-confidence. You may have been reluctant to have shown a curiosity or a knowingness about this side of sexual behaviour or you may be scared of your partner's reaction and fear rejection if you open the subject. I hope by this point you have the confidence to make such suggestions. The chances are that your partner's reaction is going to be more than positive.

The Kama Sutra suggested eight basic love-making positions, while The Perfumed Garden said there were eleven. By putting them and many other texts together, certain researchers suggest that there are well over five hundred positions, each a slight variation on the other.

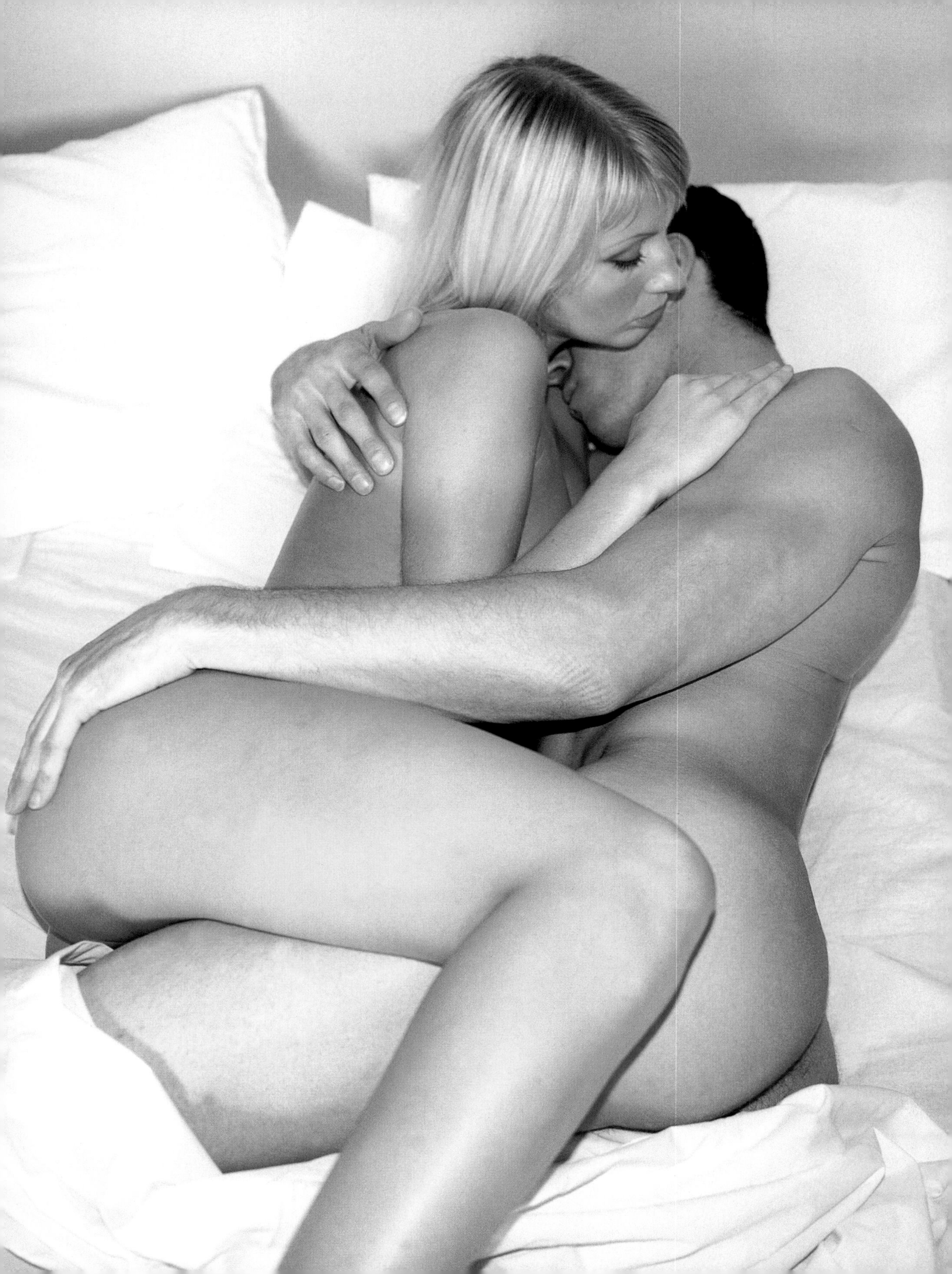

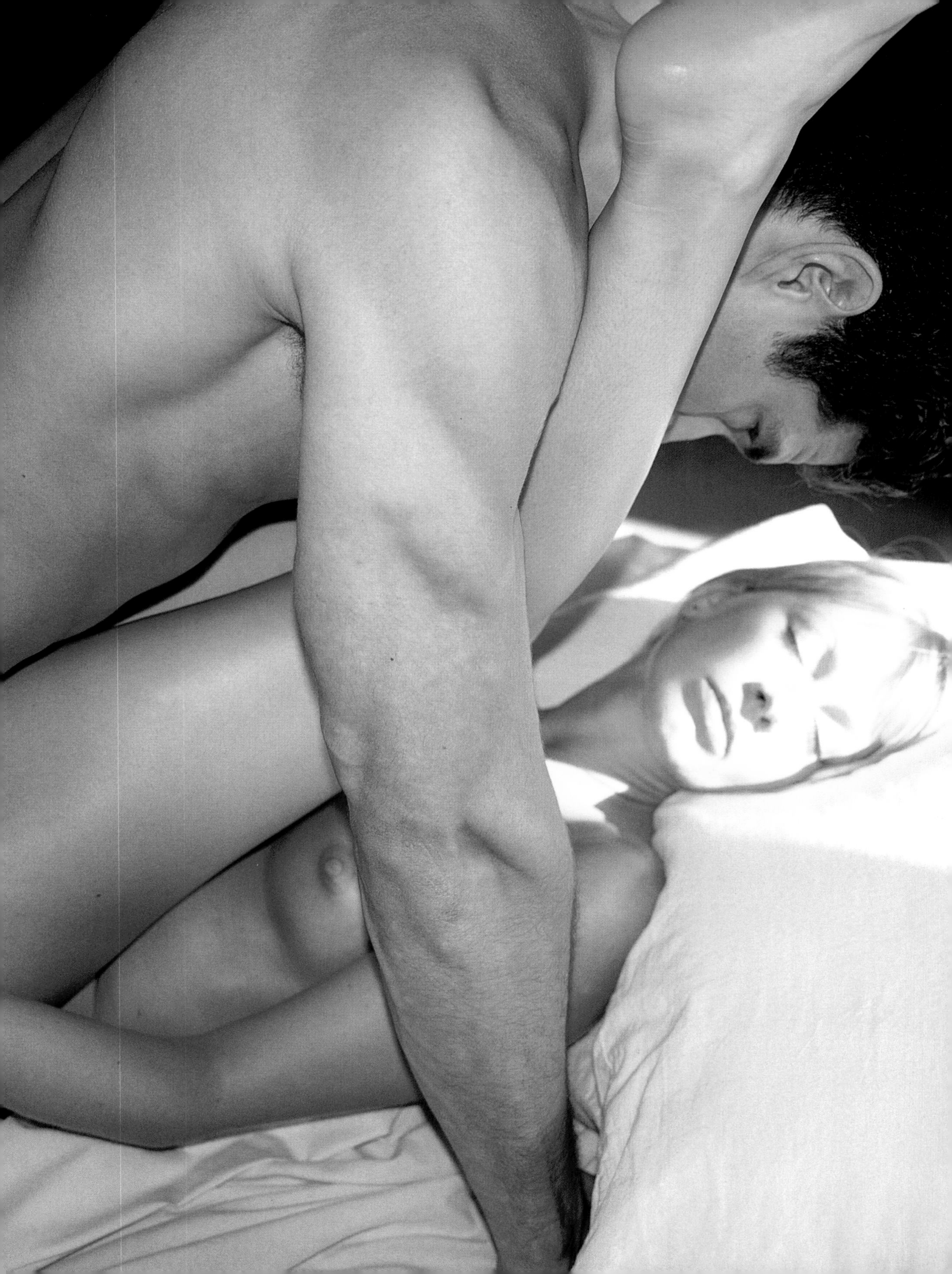

FACE TO FACE

You could start with the most popular way of having sex, which is face to face. Being eyeball to eyeball with your partner has plenty of advantages. It allows you the opportunity to gaze lovingly and intimately at each other, and to kiss mouth-to-mouth. It gives him some access to her breasts and allows both the opportunity to touch clitoris and penis before penetration, but not much after. But within the face-to-face context you have a wide variety of different positions. The most common, of course, is the so-called "missionary" position with the man lying on top of his partner, between her legs. He can support himself on his elbows and she can hold his buttocks or press down on the small of his back to steady and control the timing of his thrusts for her pleasure. There are plenty of variations on this position, where the woman can raise her legs and wrap them around her partner's waist, or she can raise them even further resting her knees against his chest or even putting her ankles on his shoulders. The only problem with the missionary position is that while it is intensely pleasurable for him it's also quite a strain making sure he doesn't press down too heavily on her breasts and ribcage. Because it may be tiring, it may hurry him along to his conclusion earlier than either of them would wish. What it may miss doing is giving sufficient stimulation to her clitoris, which is why a high proportion of women say they do not orgasm from lovemaking in this position on its own. A variation that may be enjoyable for both is when he kneels upright between her legs, or even stands. By lifting her pelvis, with his hands or by placing a pillow under her hips, he can alter the angle of entry to find a position that suits her as well as him. This position gives both of them the advantage of the man having his hands free to roam over her breasts and down to her clitoris.

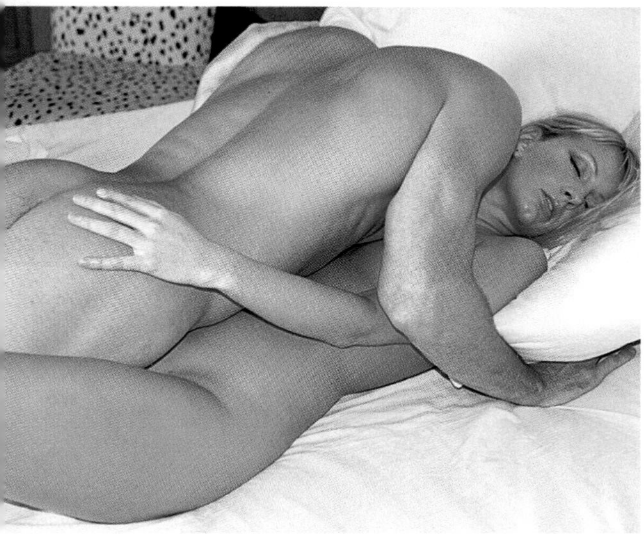

Some positions demand athleticism, others just a willingness to try something new

However, man-on-top positions leave him in the driving position. This is why the "woman-on-top", face-to-face position is top choice with many women. If you want to try woman on top and you are not sure how to suggest it to your partner, seize the opportunity when you are in a passionate clinch and simply roll over. The advantages soon become clear. With her lying or indeed sitting upward on her partner he has his hands free to stroke her body, caress her breasts and nipples and indeed to touch her clitoris gently. By taking away the need for him to support himself it also allows him to save his strength for the job in hand – most men last longer on their backs. But the main advantage of woman on top is that by having control of the speed, strength and angle of movement, women can find the point at which the clitoris is best stimulated by body-to-body contact. Women particularly find that if they ride quite high on their partner they are able to give themselves sensations that are particularly strong and satisfying.

Being face to face with your partner has plenty of advantages.

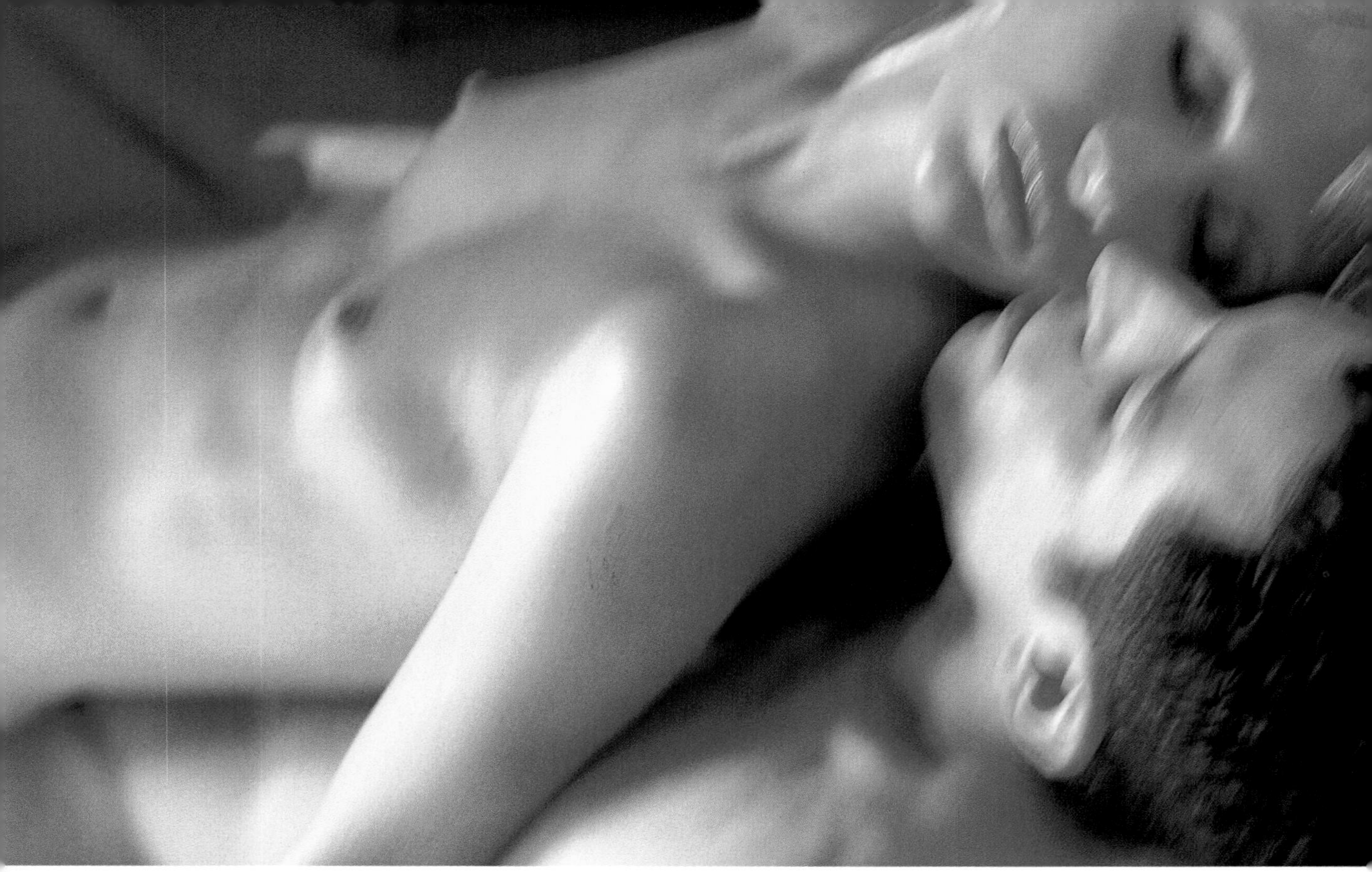

Slow and gentle sex is possible in new positions

Just as with woman on top, this is a position that gives the man staying power and the woman the majority of control and so considerably improves both their pleasure.

♦ SIDE BY SIDE

Halfway house between the two is face to face and side by side. It makes for long, slow and romantic lovemaking and you do have to hold on to make sure you don't become disconnected. There are plenty of variations on this theme. For instance, the man lying on his side with his thighs curled up and under her backside with her lying on her back with both of her legs flung over his. Full penetration is easy in this position and by moving her legs to various angles, she can have a range of different sensations.

Another variation on face to face is standing up. This is ideal for getting it together in the shower, in a lift or behind the cornflakes in the supermarket. If you are the same height you can stand genitals to genitals, but if one partner is smaller and lighter than the other they can hop up and wrap their legs around the heavier and taller partner's thighs while being held up themselves by their bottom or thighs. Needless to say, this is quite a tiring way of making love that needs plenty of practice to manage successfully. You can also face each other sitting down. You can do it on the ground, in a chair or on a bed, and it is in effect a one-to-one lap dancing display in the privacy of your own home. Just as with woman on top, this is a position that gives the man staying power and the woman the majority of control and so considerably improves both their pleasure.

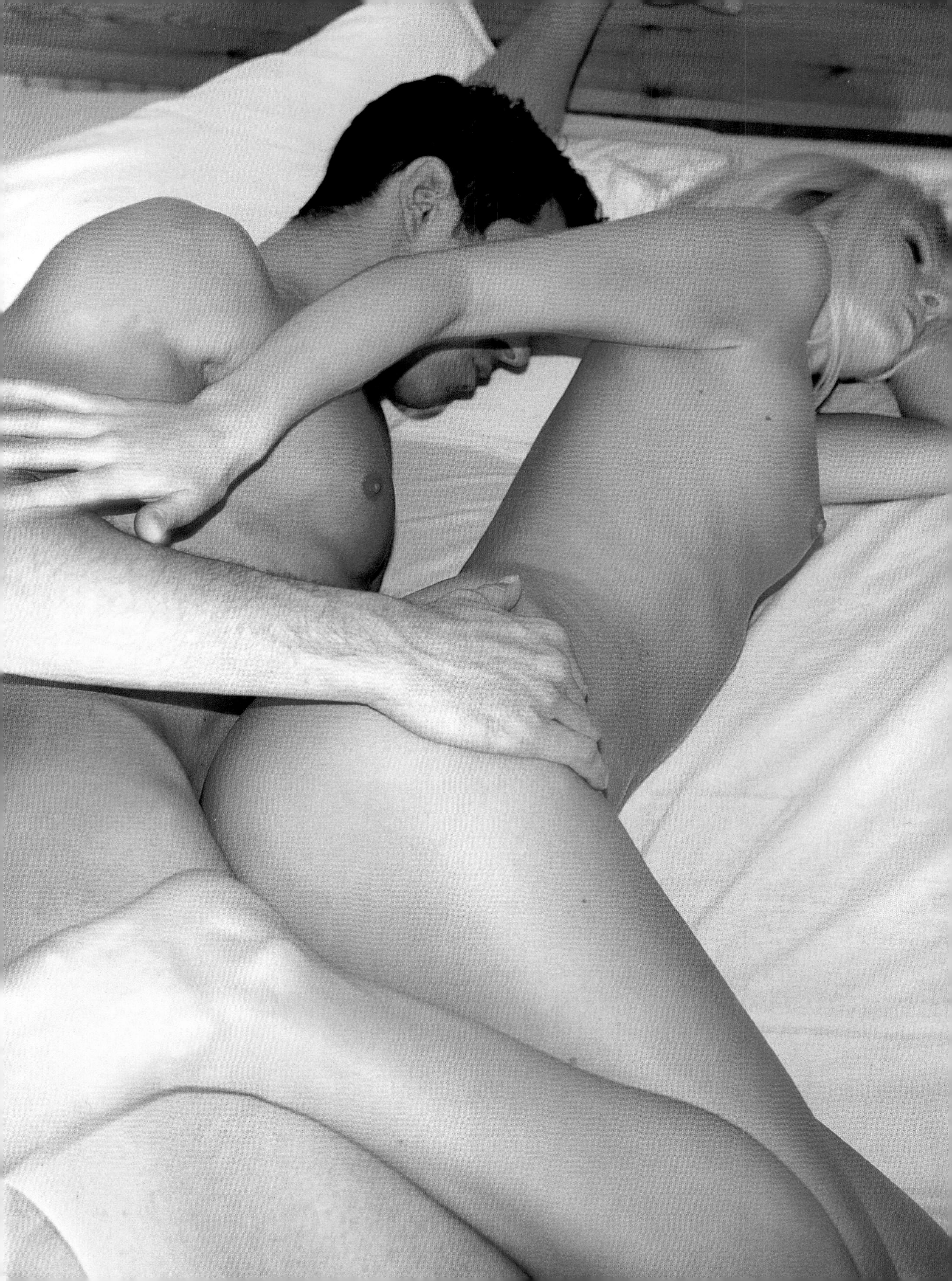

It can be the greatest compliment you can give your partner, to show them that you think they're good enough to eat.

WHAT MOST MEN WANT

Ask men what single sexual variation they'd like to add to their lovemaking, and most would vote for oral sex. It's the sex act that suffers most from fears and apprehensions, yet would often give the most satisfaction. It can be the greatest compliment you can give your partner, to show them that you think they're good enough to eat. Yet so many people fear their partners will find their private parts too unpleasant to smell, taste or look at to want to do this intimacy. In fact, most men or women are turned on by the sight, taste and smell of their partner's genitals and would be only too pleased to be allowed to show how tasty they think their lover is.

You can kiss, you can lick, you can suck or nibble. Some people prefer gentle movements, with their partner using lips and tongue to nudge them to arousal. Start off by gently running your tongue around your partner's genitals to see how they react. You may then go on to firmer attention, tonguing and nibbling or even gently nipping them. Some people like having the clitoris or glans sucked, others like their partner to blow gently on skin first made damp by licking. But, in spite of the name "blowjob", don't ever actually blow into a partner's penis or vagina. It won't be pleasurable and may cause a potentially fatal embolism or a nasty infection. You can give each other oral pleasure – him on her is called cunnilingus and her on him is called fellatio – turn and turn about. Doing it together, at the same time, is known as "69" or *soixante-neuf*. The only problem with mutual oral sex leading to climax is that it's not easy keeping up giving your partner pleasure when you, yourself, are coming. Both of you risk having your partner's interest and attention straying at the critical moment – or of having something vital bitten in the throes of excitement! You're far better off pleasuring each other to a certain point and then agreeing to let one of you go first, promising to return the compliment a few moments later.

SEX DOGGY STYLE

You don't have to be eye to eye to make love,

Many couples would love to give as well as receive oral sex

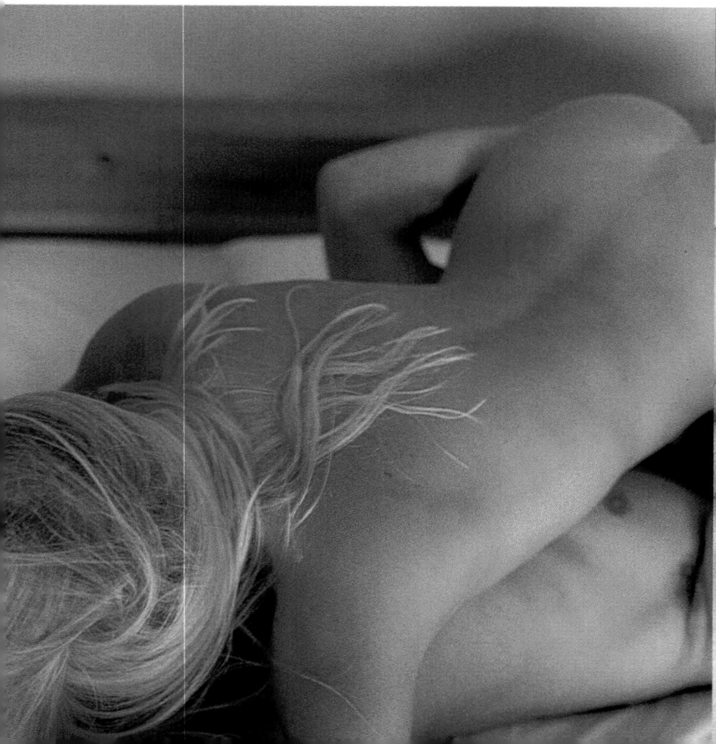
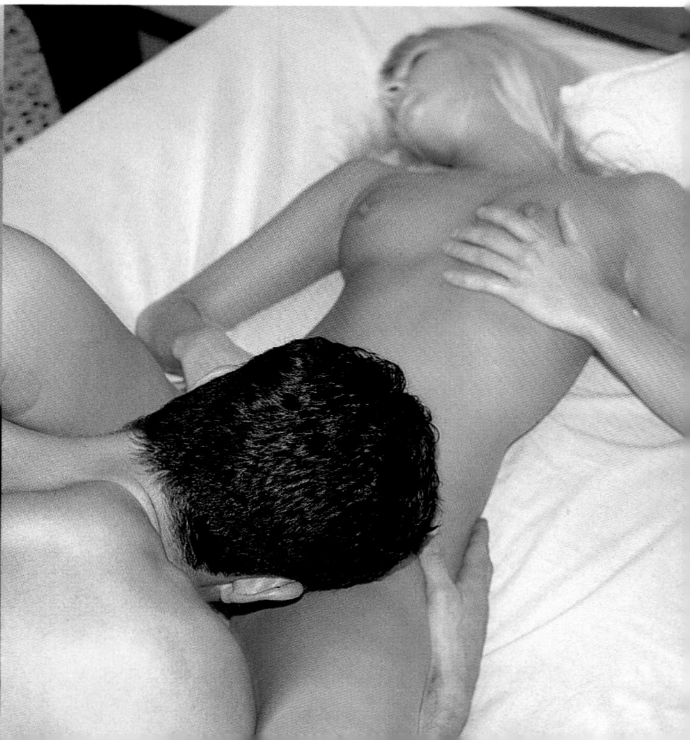

You can ring endless changes on sexual positions just by altering the disposition of your arms and legs, to suit you.

however. Indeed, our early ancestors started off having sex the same way as most of the rest of the animal kingdom, with the male entering from behind. It's a very practical position. Our forefathers needed to have sex this way so they could remain alert, one eye on the horizon, in case of danger. Today, it's know as "TV-style" and allows you to make love while both watching your favourite soap, or a raunchy film to give you ideas. Rear entry has other pluses. If he's a "bottoms man" it gives him a good view of his favourite part of his lover's body, and the opportunity to fondle her. Rear entry makes it particularly easy for either of the couple to reach and caress her clitoris and so bring her to a full orgasm. Rear entry or doggy style can also be felt to be naughty and animalistic, giving it an extra kick. You can come from behind in all sorts of ways, from standing up to lying down. A favourite position is where she lies, with her upper body propped up over pillows or cushions and her backside raised. He kneels between her legs and enters her. But he can also stand behind as she leans over the side of a bed or chair, or hold her legs up as he stands between them. You can sit, she either sitting on his lap with her back fully to him or turned halfway round, one arm around his neck. Finally, you can have rear-entry sex lying side by side, spoon-fashion.

You can ring endless changes on sexual positions just by altering the disposition of your arms and legs, to suit you. Start off by finding a basic position that appeals to you – say, face to face and woman on top. You may commence by having her lie on his chest, supported on her elbows and with her legs on either side of his thighs. Experiment by having her rearing up on her hands. See what happens when she shifts one or both legs to lie inside his thighs. And how about sitting up, and bringing her knees up? How does it feel if she crouches, and then turns so she faces his feet? You may collapse in giggles, or get stuck or come adrift. It doesn't matter. Just keep trying out different ways of feeling good and seeing how the two of you can ring the changes on fitting together and making each other feel good.

Naughty but nice – doggy sex has always been popular

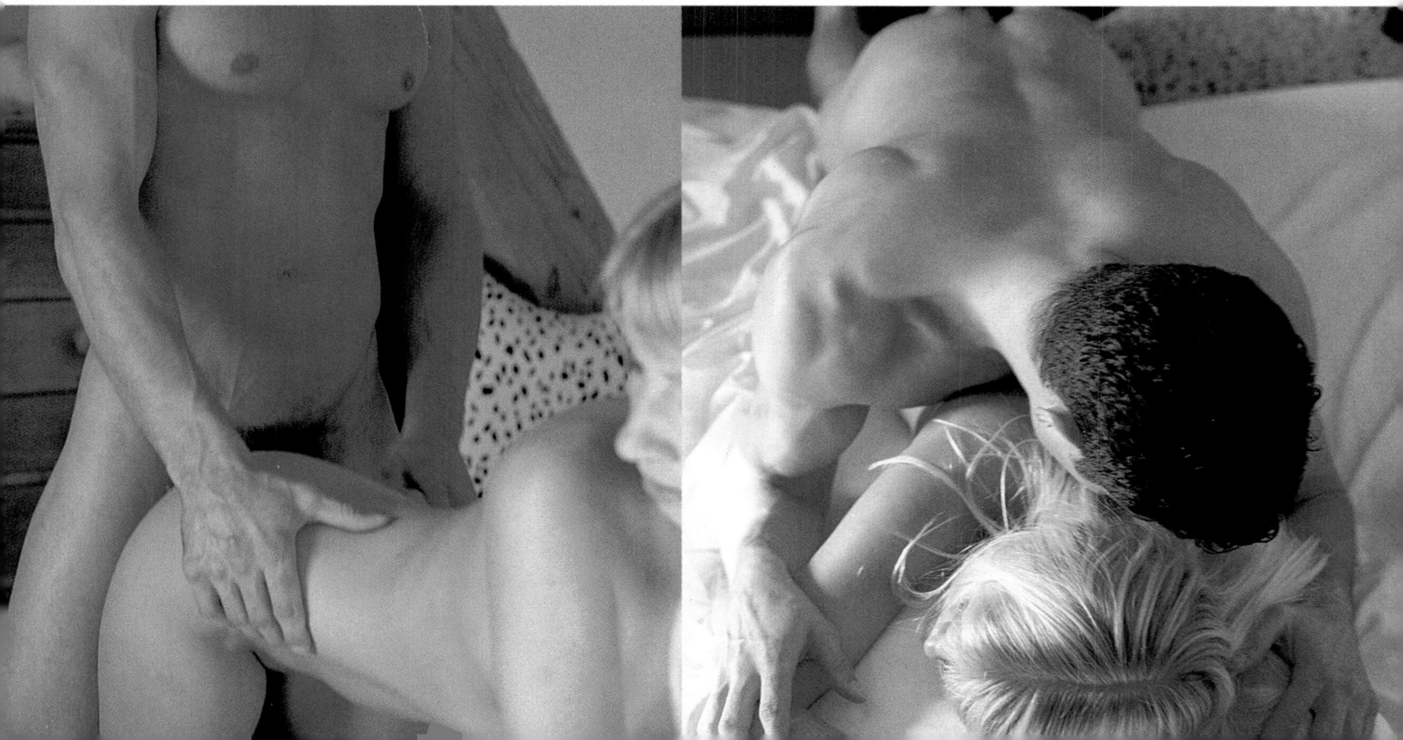

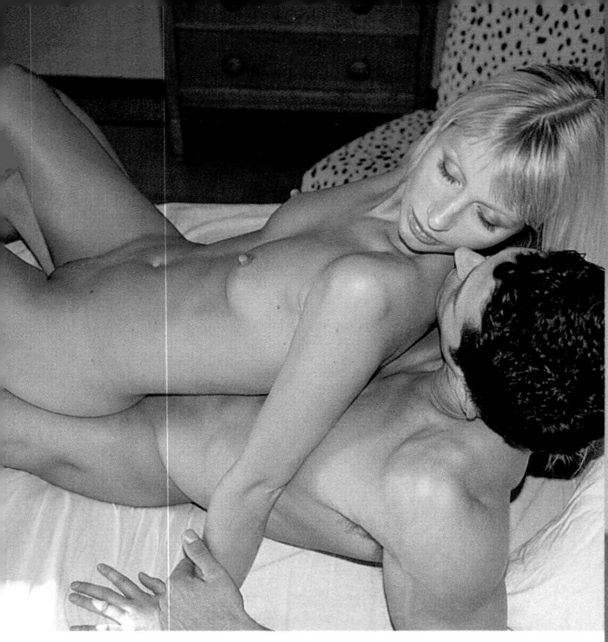

You can ring endless changes

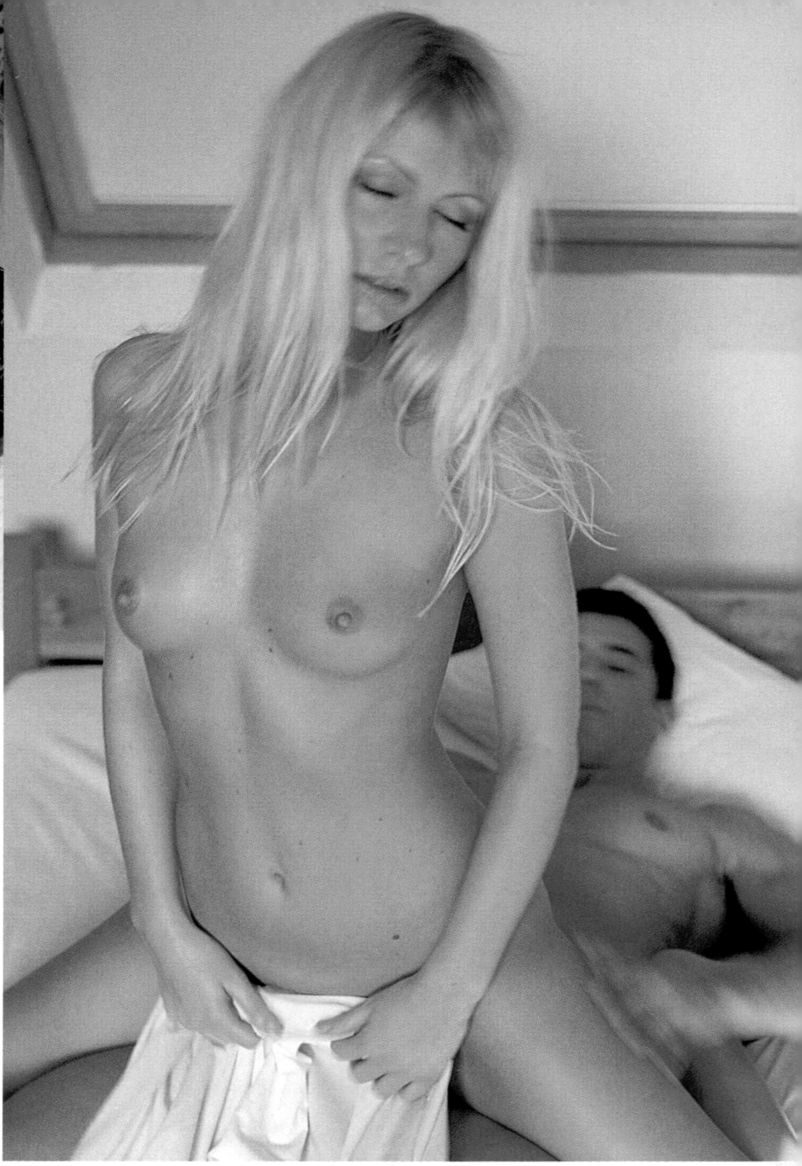

Experimenting will help you find new positions

TRY SOMETHING NEW

If you want to experiment with some new sexual positions but are a bit unclear as to how to start or what to try, have a go with a fantasy game that could get you swinging from the chandelier. The problem is that, in spite of there being well over 500 (some say, 521 to be precise) different positions for making love we all tend to fall back on the good old "missionary" position. It's a pity, because other positions have a lot to recommend them. To make love in a way that truly satisfies both parties, you need to fulfil certain conditions. He needs to have the head of his penis gripped and stimulated. She needs to have her clitoris massaged and caressed. Both find arousal aided by having the obvious erogenous areas such as lips, nipples and the inside of thighs and the less obvious ones such as earlobes, necks, and backs stroked. As we've already pointed out, man on top is probably the worst position of all to fulfil all these. His penis may get all the attention it needs but the angle is often wrong for her clitoris to be stimulated to her fulfilment. This is why so many women find intercourse curiously unsatisfying even though masturbation hits the spot for them. If you want to find an over-abundance of exciting ways of pleasing each other, you need to be more adventurous in the ways you go at it. So use this game to try woman on top, or sitting face to face on a bed, the woman sitting on her partner's lap. Have a go at experimenting with standing, face to face or with the man entering his partner from behind. Or try lying side by side, her back to his front in the spoon position. See how, in many of these positions, both partners' hands may be free to manipulate nipples, breasts, clitoris and testicles. But getting started on trying something new can be daunting. You may feel uneasy or confused, scared to show inexperience and not sure how you may be able to manage. This game is a good way of getting over the initial uncertainty.

SEXUAL ATHLETES

Imagine yourselves to be sexual athletes, representing your country in the World Sex Cup. You've both trained for years to get to this peak of athletic prowess and sexual skill. There are, however, new positions being devised all the time and you need to allow for a little clumsiness as you try them out. Practice makes perfect, however – you just need plenty of practice. You know that the more unusual the sexual position you try, the higher the points you'll get. But you also get points for style and content, and for sexual satisfaction, so you need to find a new position that works for both of you. Talk over the sexual positions you may have used to make love together – you may have tried woman on top, doggy fashion, standing up or you may not yet have ventured past man on top. Whatever, anything you've done so far is off limits now as being far too boring to earn points. Think about sexual positions you've heard about – standing, sitting, from behind, woman on top. You could also consider "69", with both of you giving the other oral sex, or trying it turn and turn about. You're about to start an hour-long training session, so get to it! You'll need a towel and energy drinks to keep you going through all that hot and sweaty work. Consider the advice given by the *Kama Sutra*, that there are eight basic positions for making love, and by *The Perfumed Garden*, which says there are eleven. What both agree is that there are literally hundreds of possible variations. You can ring eternal changes by shifting your bodies, bending or straightening legs, sitting up, leaning over or by supporting yourself on elbows, arms or knees. You can make a difference by using pillows, walls, chairs, washing machines to sit on or drape yourself across or prop you up. The ancients gave the sexual positions they described the most wonderful names, such as "Two Fishes Side By Side" or "Cat And Mouse Share A Hole". Find your own variations, and come up with your own name to describe it. Play this fantasy game when there is international gymnastics, athletics or ice skating on the television. Use the commentary, the marks and the applause as yours. Of course, when you're really experienced, try it to the Tour de France – all fourteen days of it!

Using a fantasy game as a way of beginning to try out new positions can be a fun way of livening up your sex life. Anne and Tom had wanted to be more adventurous in bed for some time but never quite got round to it. Theirs was a second relationship for both of them. Anne had been married to a boy she had met at school, and Tom was the second person she'd ever had sex with. Tom wasn't much more experienced. Their sex life was happy in that they were madly in love with each other. But the extent of both their sexual repertoires was man on top, with a hesitant bit of oral sex. Both longed to try out the positions they'd read about and seen in films and books, but neither felt either confident enough to suggest it or competent enough to try. One night, watching athletics on late-night television in bed, Tom misheard a commentary. They both collapsed in giggles as he then put a sexual slant on everything said. They imagined the rest of the programme as a Sexual Olympics and started suiting their own actions to what the commentator seemed to be saying was going on. Egged on by descriptions, such as "look at the height he's got into that" or "just see the way she puts a curve into her stroke" Anne and Tom had their first training session. Emboldened by this first attempt, they went on to experience more and more exotic sexual positions and eventually bought a copy of the *Kama Sutra*, to see which they hadn't found out for themselves.

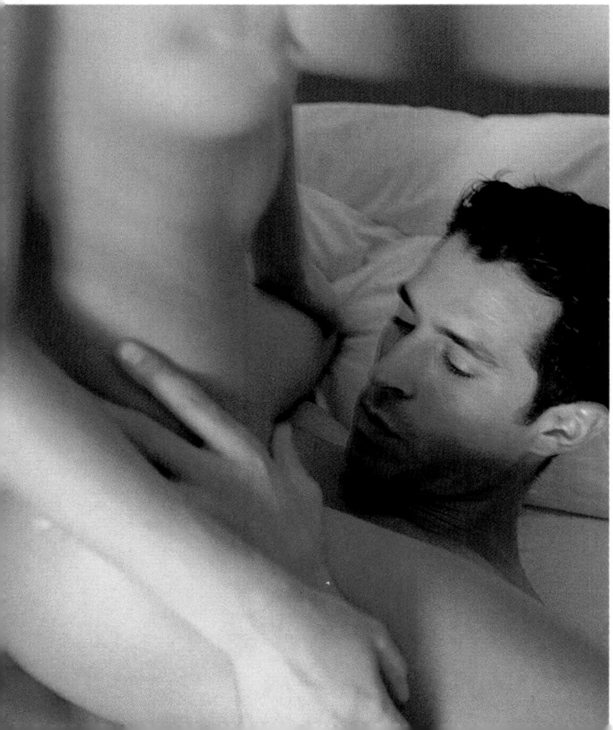

Most men would be pleased to taste their partner's body

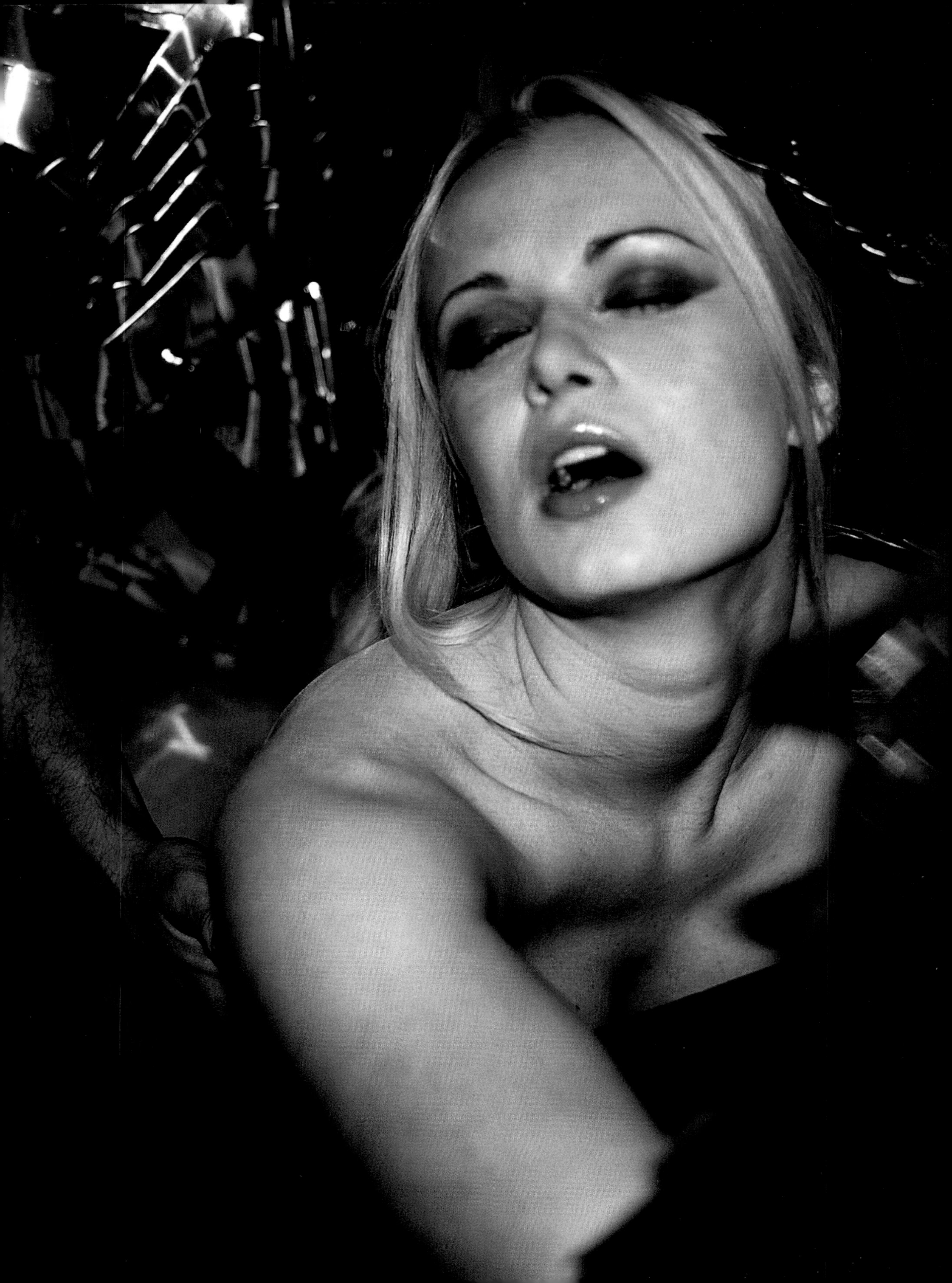

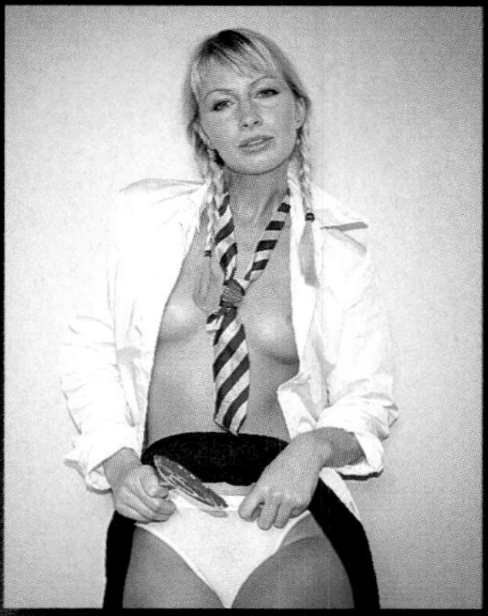

Chapter 7

BE MY FANTASY

Everyone has sexual fantasies. You may call them wool-gathering, daydreams or wishful thinking, but whatever label you put on them, they are a universal part of sexuality. And they're not exactly new, either. Cleopatra is said to have seduced Marc Antony by sweeping him away on her luxury barge where she was dressed as Venus, and surrounded with attendants got up as cupids and nymphs.

Emperor Nero would persuade the high-born ladies of his court to act as prostitutes in an imaginary brothel so he could live out one of his fantasies. Marie Antoinette got off by imagining herself as a milkmaid, frolicking with King Louis in a specially-constructed luxury milking parlour with marble milking stall and gold pails. Closer to our own times, J. Edgar Hoover, the all-powerful head of the FBI, is reported to have found his escape from the affairs of state by dressing up in women's clothes and playing out his own sexual fantasies on a regular basis.

We tend, however, to feel that sexual fantasy is largely a male thing – that particular element of Cleo's and Marie's behaviour has usually been played down and misrepresented. Some men find it rather disconcerting to learn that women are now accepted as

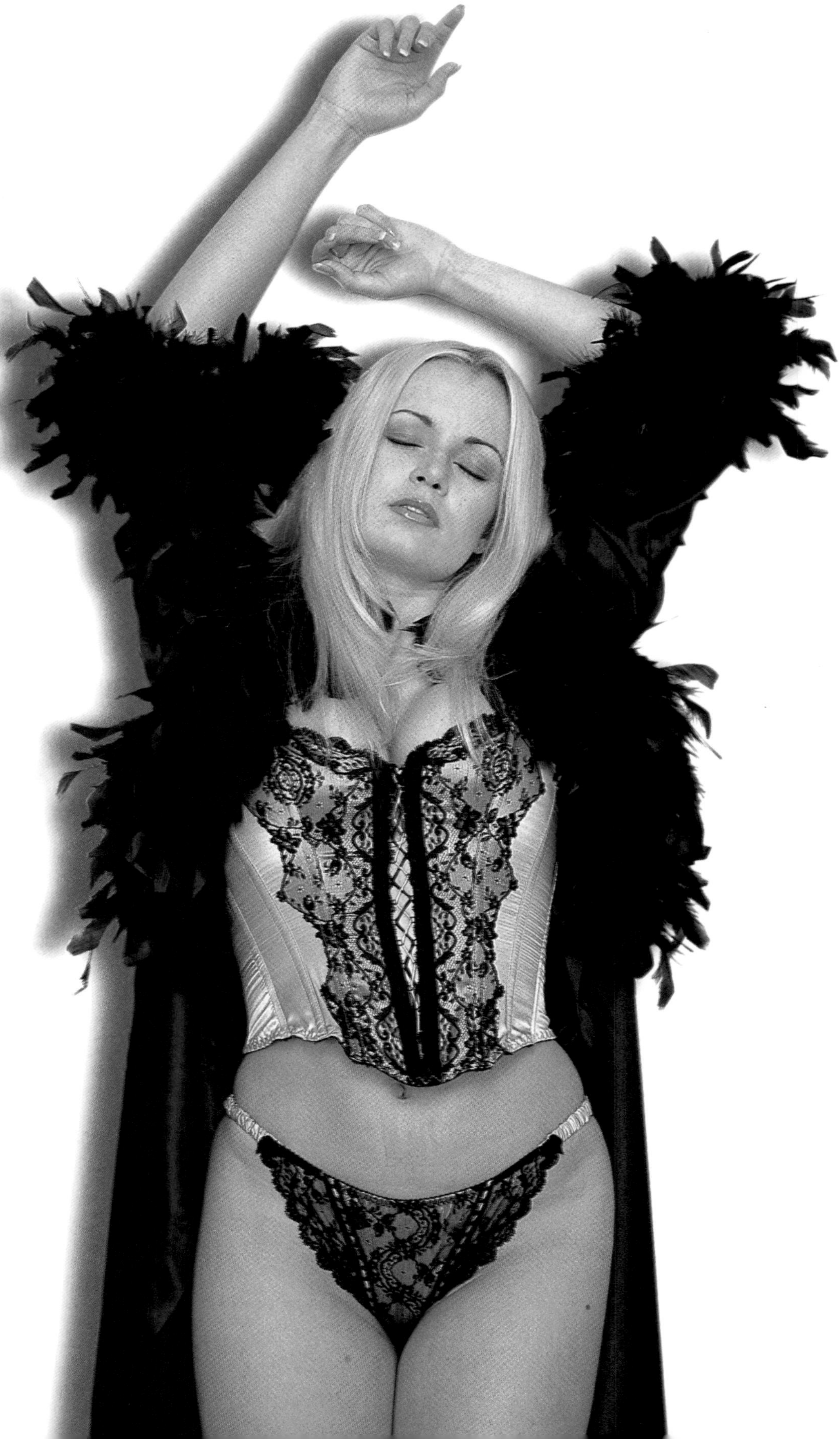

having as rich and raunchy a fantasy life as they do. Sadly, there are still some people who seem to feel that women don't or shouldn't have sexual fantasies, and this has led many women to feel quite ashamed of doing so. In fact, when it comes to fantasies, and especially fantasizing about sex, women and men have far more similarities than differences. It's now generally accepted that almost three-quarters of both men and women fantasize quite specifically to increase their excitement while having sex and to make sex more satisfying. Women have even moved on to the stage where they actually use their fantasies to make themselves rich and famous. After all, what are today's women writers of "bodice-rippers" and "sex-and-shopping" blockbusters doing but putting elaborate female sexual fantasies into words on paper?

SEXUAL FANTASIES AND GUILT

Even with all these examples of others having fantasies, you may not be prepared to admit to having them yourself, especially if your upbringing left the unspoken lesson that sex is rather dirty and frightening and sexual feelings and sexual thoughts are something to feel guilty about. Some of us have been unlucky enough to be subjected to the kind of thinking that's hardly changed since medieval times. Then it was believed that evil spirits or demons – incubi and succubi – would visit people in their sleep and seduce them against their will. These beliefs made it very hard for people to accept their own harmless sexual fantasies and, rather than enjoying them, they would feel guilty and sinful. An elaborate mythology was erected around the belief that dreams came from outside rather than from a person's own thoughts. While incubi and succubi are no longer with us, we can still share an almost medieval fear about many of our sexual feelings and find it difficult to accept them.

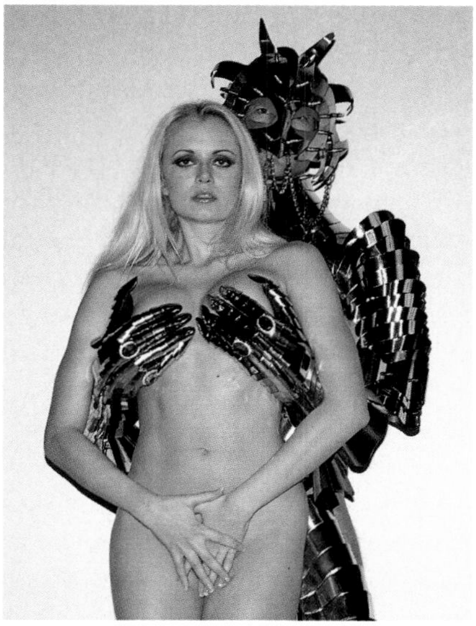

Sexual fantasies are harmless

But whether we feel guilt about our sexual fantasies or accept and get pleasure from them, the actual reasons why we do fantasize will be the same. What we are really doing is extending a technique we all use in our childhood and making it meet our adult needs. As children, we would act out in games or in our imagination the things that happened to us or that we had seen, and run through and try for size our feelings about them. The fantasy and playtime could give us the opportunity to take charge and do things our own way, or experiment to make an event run a different course or have a different ending to what had happened in real life. We can carry this over into our later life, for fun or when we are feeling confused, powerless or under someone else's control. This is why fantasy, and especially sexual fantasy, is so important and so powerful. It can let you imagine that your life, and especially your love life, is satisfying and going the way you want it, even if the reality is very different. But sexual fantasy isn't only a form of redress. Even if you have a wildly passionate and happy sexual relationship, sexual fantasy can help you put the cherry on the icing on the cake.

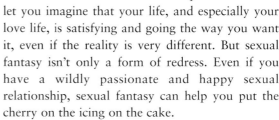

If you can't make love with the one you love, you can fantasize and imagine them there while you pleasure yourself.

♦ VIRTUAL REALITY SEX

Sexual fantasy can give you a partner when for some reason or other you don't have access to the real thing. If you can't make love with the one you love, you can fantasize and imagine them there while you pleasure yourself. Similarly, there can be times when having sex together doesn't work out – because one or both of you is ill or tired, because of the infirmities of old age or because finding time to be together in private is hard. You may also be on your own, temporarily or permanently, because of divorce or death or when one of you is away for work reasons. On all these occasions you can use sexual fantasy and dreams – of your partner or of another person – to meet your sexual needs at the time. Even if you have none of these complications, there can still be disagreement between partners about how much sex they should be having. The "not getting enough" partner can then use fantasy to fill in the gaps left by the more sexually temperate other half. Fantasy can also fill in any other gaps, such as having sexual variations that one partner might not be too keen on. You could even extend this "virtual reality" approach to having an affair, without actually committing adultery.

Sexual fantasy can be the solution when you don't want to have sex with your partner, at all or at a particular time, but feel unable to say no. Then, you replace them in your mind with someone who does excite or please you, or use fantasy in some other way to make things more acceptable or exciting. It can also be a safety valve to relieve any tensions or worries you might have about yourself or your sexual behaviour. In your own mind, and under your control, no sexual partner is going to laugh at your body, criticize your technique or question your tastes.

Whatever way you use fantasy – just for fun, as a safe environment to try things out, as a way of rehearsing what you might want to do, or trying something like rape, which is exciting in theory but which you would never want to experience in reality – its undeniable advantage is that you are in absolute control. You could say that sexual fantasy is like the perfect film, and you are the producer, the director, scriptwriter, casting agent and camera operator. Every scene, every last detail begins and ends as you decide – without the guilt, anxieties and embarrassments that such scenarios could provoke in real life.

♦ MALE AND FEMALE SEXUAL FANTASIES

As has been said, in both real sex and fantasy sex, men and women seem to have more common elements than dissimilar ones. Any differences in the sexual fantasy area reflect the way we see women in society rather than our real feelings under the surface. For instance, men tend to fantasize about things they have already done, reliving a particularly good sexual encounter or something they've actually seen in a magazine or on the screen. Women tend to be more imaginative, coming up with things they haven't yet tried or even seen. This probably reflects the fact that in real relationships it is the man who suggests or chooses what a couple does. Women are often too shy to make suggestions for fear of being accused of being too experienced or too "knowing", both of which are seen to be acceptable characteristics for men and unacceptable ones for women. So women are far more likely to have unfulfilled desires than men. Men may also be more prone to fantasize about specific sexual acts, while women may be more likely to imagine a whole scenario involving love, romance and strong feelings. But having said that, many men do dream about love and romance and many women do dream of lust.

The "not getting enough" partner can then use fantasy to fill in the gaps left by the more sexually temperate other half.

The key element to all sexual-fantasy sex is that it is fantasy. Daydreaming that you would like to be gang-banged, have gay sex or be hung from the ceiling by your better bits does not mean that you might actually enjoy the reality. It merely means that you enjoy the thought and that your thoughts are your business and not open to anyone else's judgement. You can keep your fantasies strictly in your mind, and use them as a private video show to spice up your imagination, either when you're on your own or when you and your partner are making love. You can go one step further and tell your partner what your fantasies are. Some couples find it really does enliven their shared love-making if each talk the other through what is going on in their minds. But just as many couples get a kick out of going the whole hog and acting out their fantasies. To do so, you need to share and discuss your ideas and agree to play them for real.

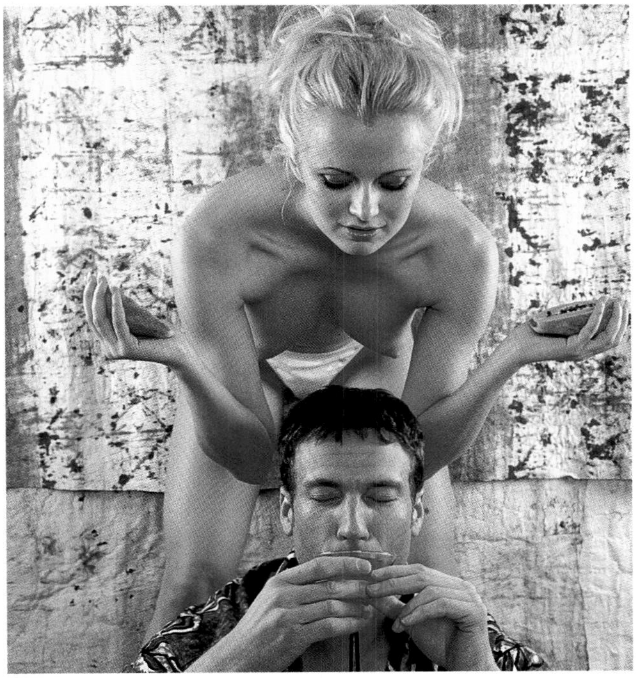

Transport yourselves into your dreams

POPULAR SEXUAL FANTASIES

So, what are the most popular fantasies and why are they there? The most common fantasy, for both men and women, is something involving sex with a current partner. This may seem most unadventurous – after all, what's the point of dreaming about the person you're actually having sex with? But the reason is that we largely use the fantasy to get it absolutely right and to imagine having wonderful sex without all the niggles, lumps, bumps and irritations that can intrude on the real thing. We may imagine having sex with them at home, in our own double bed, or in some location around the house that we might like to try but have been too shy to suggest, such as on the kitchen table, on the patio or on the front doorstep. More often, we dream about having sex in a perfectly ideal situation. This often means imagining being with your partner in an exotic location.

EXOTIC EROTIC

Having sex somewhere different, foreign, even outlandish is a favourite daydream for most of us. The reason is that being away from home often releases us from stresses and restraints. It works in reality, when you go away on holiday. Being surrounded by strangers with none of the friends, family or neighbours to tut-tut and carry tales, many of us throw away our inhibitions and act in ways we'd never dream of doing at home. We get drunk, dance on tables, flirt outrageously with our own partners or fall in love with and make love to people we've only just met. But it's not just a question of no longer

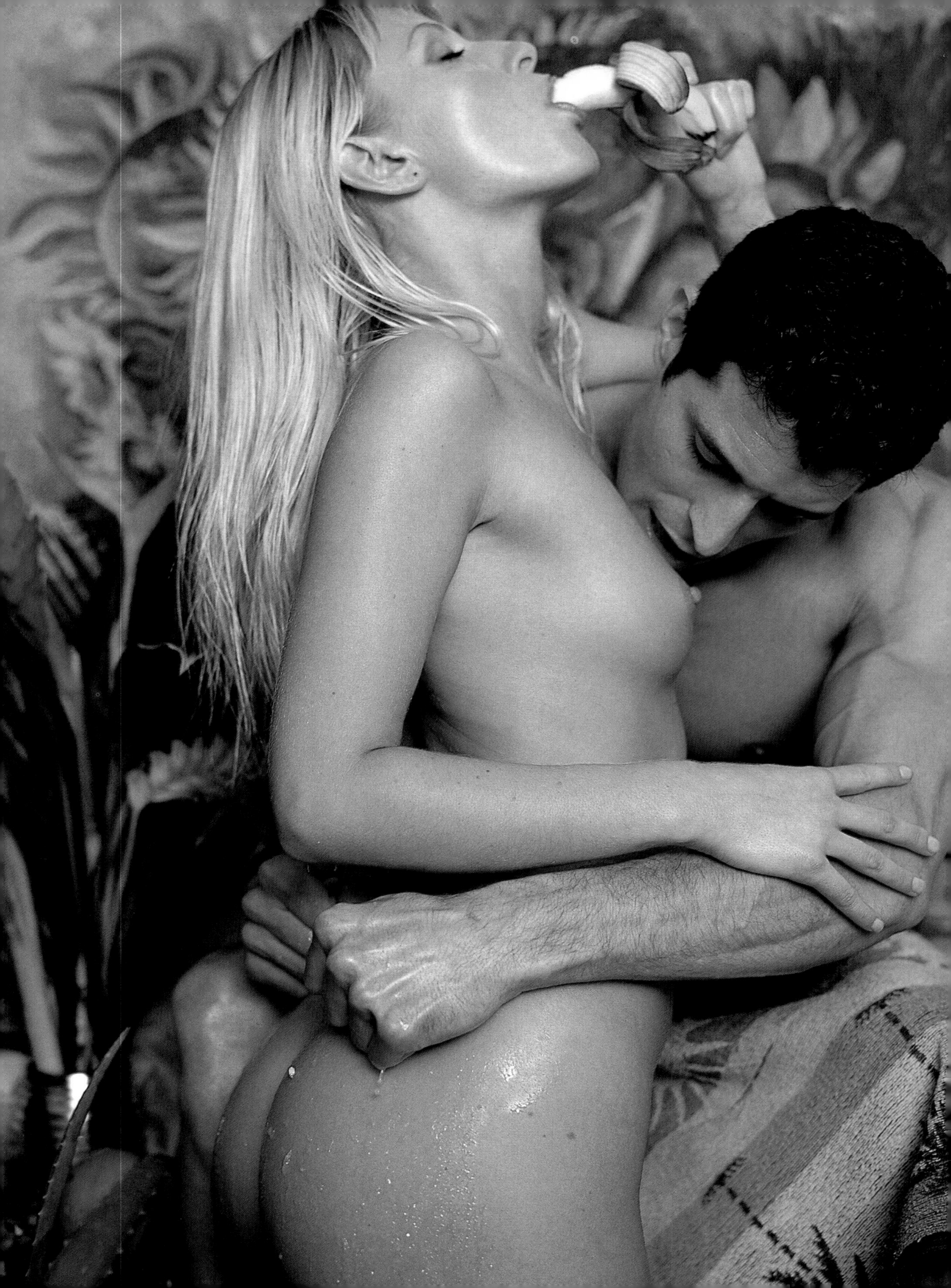

having to worry about our reputation. It's also because we feel reality has taken a holiday, too. Back home, you wouldn't just be afraid of what people would think or say, you'd be scared of the consequences. On holiday, you tend to feel they don't exist – as if a pregnancy or a sexual infection won't know where you live once you've gone home! Another reason is that we tend to feel they do it differently and far more sexily abroad, so throwing caution and inhibitions to the winds is only following local customs.

SETTING OURSELVES FREE

You can use all this to cut loose in a sexual fantasy. Most of us need a way of feeling permitted to access our deepest, most secret and passionate desires. Imagining yourself in your dream place, far away from home and all its restraints, can do the trick. Your personal fantasy could involve a Caribbean beach, for example. If you would like to give this a try, set the scene by arranging plants and vases of flowers around the living room to mimic the jungle edge. Turn up the heating and if you've a sunlamp, put it on. Lay out a beach towel on the floor or over a sofa, to stand in for a sun lounger. Bring the exotic to life and into your home by conjuring up unfamiliar scents and flavours. If you're setting the scene on a desert island, burn some incense. Mix up the sort of cocktail you only drink on holiday – a jug of Sangria, a tall glass of Tequila Sunset or Rum Punch. Set your exotic drink by the side of your towel or lounger along with a bowl of exotic fruit and bottle of suntan oil. You could also add a feather – it should be from the sort of parrots you'd find flying around your desert island idyll but one from a peacock or pheasant or even a chicken will do fine. Dress yourselves in brief swimming gear – a bikini for her, a thong for him. Close your eyes and imagine you've flown out the previous night and have just woken up to Paradise. You've wandered out of your luxury hotel room, strolled down the beach and have found a private area, obviously set up for your delight. You are sitting in the shade of the palms when you realize you're the only people there. You could almost believe you're castaways, shipwrecked on a deserted island.

TAKE IT FROM HERE

Start the action by offering to spread suntan oil on your partner, asking that they do the same to you. You could use dialogue you've agreed before, or improvise as you like. Perhaps she says, "There's no reason to even keep our thongs on – here's the chance to get an all-over tan." He says, "Sure, but I've got bits that have never been seen by the sun! If we're going to lie here starkers, that means we need to make sure every last inch of skin is covered and protected by suntan cream." Spread the oil or suntan cream all over each other, making sure to pay attention to every last bit. You'll raise the temperature if you give each other a running commentary as you do it, saying exactly where you intend to rub the lotion and where you think you still need to be covered. "You need some here, on your nipples. Is that OK? Let me just smooth some here, on the inside of your thigh. Am I tickling you?" Don't forget the cold drinks and fruit. One of you could take a drink to cool down, and trickle a little on your partner's belly or down a cleavage. "Here, this will cool you down," you could say as you lick it off. The contrast between the heat and the cold can have parts of your body stand up to attention. Or you could cut open a peach and let the juice drip down your partner's legs,

"...in some places, it's considered really bad luck to make love indoors. Outdoor sex is the only acceptable way so we're only doing the done thing!"

Left: Imagining yourself in a dream place can spice up your sex life as you throw away your inhibitions

and clean it off with your tongue. Or slowly drop grapes, one by one, into your partner's open mouth. Imagine you can feel the heat and pretend it's almost too hot to do anything as energetic as make love – you might tickle each other with a feather, found on the beach. But mostly it's better, surely, just to smooth on the oil and lie there, enjoying the scenery. But as you stroke and caress each other's bodies, the fact that there is no one else in sight means you can fulfil a life-long wish – to make love on the sand. "Did you know," she could say, "in some places, it's considered really bad luck to make love indoors. Outdoor sex is the only acceptable way so we're only doing the done thing!"

If your fantasy place is a snow-covered chalet in a mountain retreat with a roaring log fire, lay out a shaggy or fleecy rug in front of your heat source. To bring your mountain lodge to mind, burn pine or cedarwood incense and brew up some mulled wine or *Gluwein* to drink, or make up mugs of creamy hot chocolate or hot buttered punch. Have some lotion on hand "to drive away the chill". Instead of a feather with which to tickle your partner, have a fur or fleece glove or scarf with which to tease and tantalize them. Set the scene. You've just come in out of a blizzard, frozen to the bone and in wet clothes. "The best way to warm up is to strip out of these, and rub each other all over with a nice, warm towel. You'll catch your death if you don't get some feeling back into those toes. Here, let me rub some lotion over you to bring life and feeling back into you." You'll need to stroke and stimulate every last inch of skin to make sure every bit is safe, and spill warm chocolate on each other to make sure you're toasty warm. "Is this bit still frozen? Just show me which bits on you are still in need of being warmed up! Just touch me here, I'm all pins and needles from the cold."

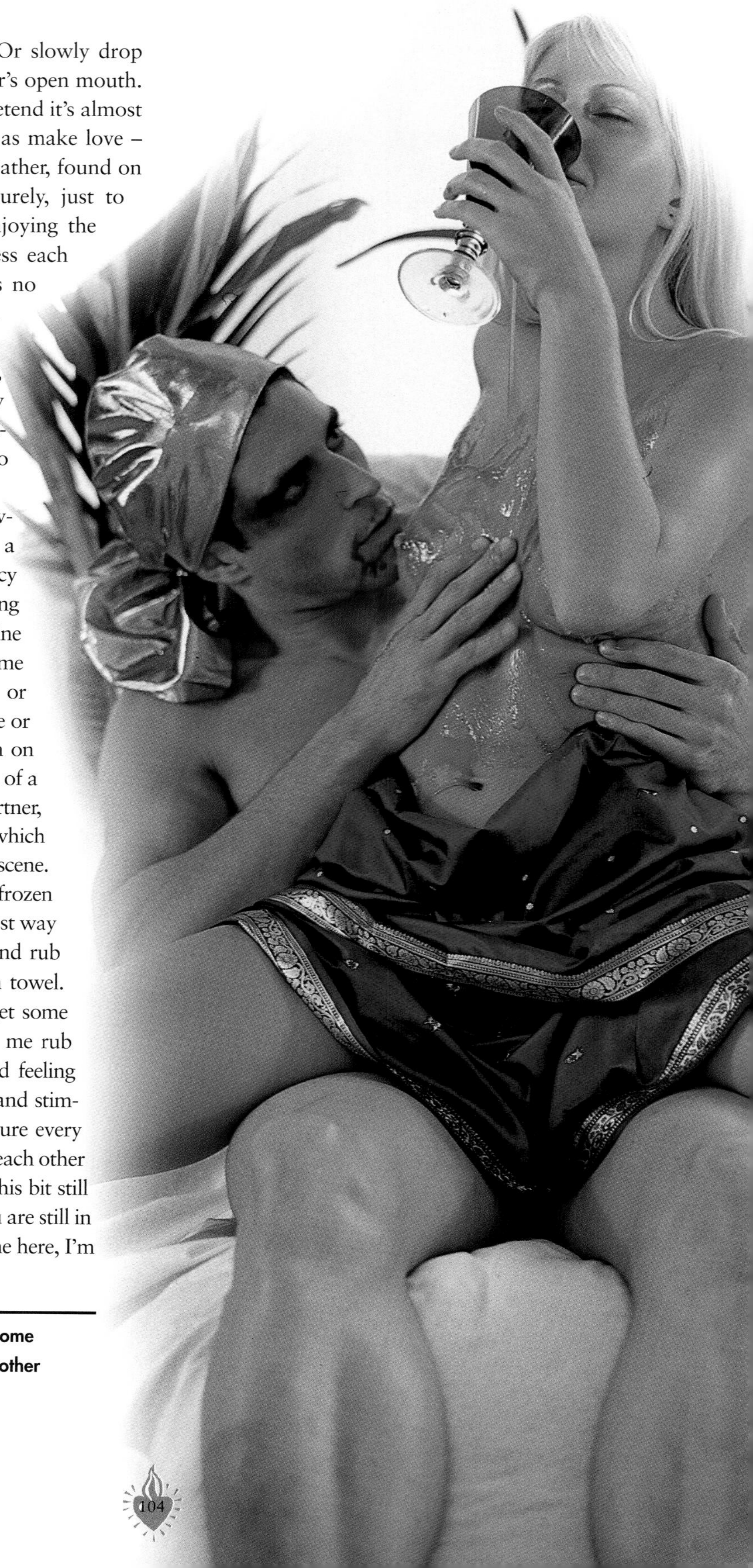

An Arabian Nights feast with a handsome prince can soon have you eating each other

THE BENEFITS OF SEXUAL FANTASIES

Imagining yourselves transported to your favourite location can revive a flagging relationship. Deedee and Nico had been together for eight years when they went to counselling for help. The trigger was a holiday with friends in Malta. Having not had sex for six months, they found themselves making every excuse under the sun to sneak away to their room. Once there, instead of having the "only when the lights are out, under the covers" sort of sex they'd been having at home, they were practically swinging from the chandelier. Once home, they let weeks drift by before making love again and when sex did happen, both were dreadfully disappointed to find that it was routine and boring again. Neither could quite put a finger on what was wrong, what made the difference and what to do about it. Talking it over with some help, they realized that holidays in the sun spelled out freedom, sex and romance to them both. Life at home meant restrictions. The stresses of running a busy work and home life left them with little time or energy to concentrate on each other or their sex life. They wanted and needed to bring some of their holiday relaxation home but found it hard. Their counsellor suggested exploring what made holiday sex so good by using their imaginations and playing a fantasy sex game. Imagining themselves back in their Maltese villa allowed both of them to recreate the feelings that went with that particular time and place. Once they'd done it at home in a fantasy game a few times, they found they could be uninhibited and sensual together without pretending. Mind you, they also discovered that playing games added such a spice to their sex life, they hardly looked back.

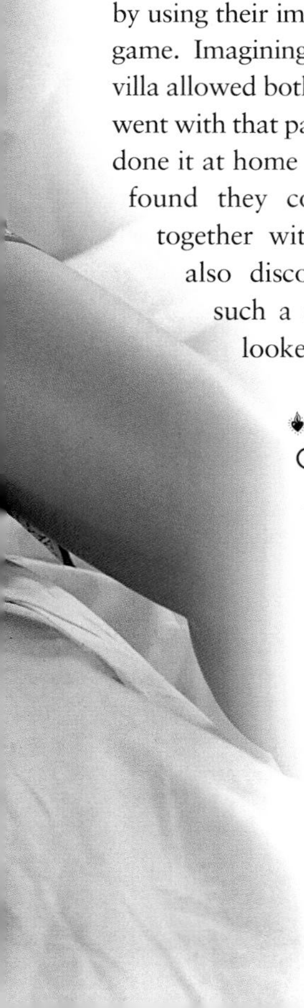

SOME DAY MY PRINCE WILL COME

A variation on this theme is when you travel in time as well as place. You may like to add a historical spin on your fantasy setting or add another element, such as bringing in the seductive power of food and drink. Food and drink often enhance sex. A candlelit dinner isn't only romantic because your companion looks enticing in the flickering light. It's because, as you nibble, lick and slurp your food, both of you send the message that you would like to do the same to various parts of your lover's body. And some foods are inextricably linked to sex. We believe that many edibles have the power to affect our sex lives, by increasing our sexual desire or sexual capabilities. Long, penis-shaped foods, such as bananas or asparagus, and substances such as powdered rhino horn, are reputed to give men vigorous erections and make them potent. Figs, which look like the inside of the vulva, and oysters, which have an intimate feminine odour, are supposed to put both sexes in the mood for love, as is chocolate. Hot, spicy foods such as curry and chilli are reputed to raise the temperature, put us in mind of aromatic and sweaty encounters and to heat the sexual organs directly. And, of course, drinks such as champagne have always had a sexy reputation. The bubbles get up your nose, loosen your inhibitions and put you in the mood for other frothy explosions.

Eat your way through the food, quaff the drink and devour each other as well. You know you're good enough to eat.

All this explains why a very popular fantasy is having sex in a Regency or "Arabian Nights" palace, with your prince or princess, surrounded by decadent luxury. Set the scene with a shopping trip, stocking up with as much of the special foods and drink as you can afford. Prepare your room as a harem or a palace. Turn the lights low, and have the room lit by candles on every surface. Pile the bed or floor with cushions or pillows and spread plates, bowls, bottles and glasses full of food and drink all around you. Dress yourselves in sumptuous, richly coloured and textured clothing. If you're going for the Eastern style, wear caftans or kimonos, or tie and drape sarongs or silk-type scarves over yourself. Start the action by imagining you're both sensualists, about to embark on an evening of voluptuous pleasure with all the time in the world. Anything that feels good and pleases your partner too is allowed. You're going to eat your way through the food, quaff the drink and devour each other as well. You know you're good enough to eat, and your partner is about to prove it. Slowly and seductively, feed titbits to each other. Pick up a peach, a fig, a spear of asparagus or bar of crumbly chocolate as is appropriate and lick, suck and nibble, saying, "This reminds me of you. Is this what you'd like me to do to you?" Dribble spoonfuls of wine, cream or ice cream on each other and lick it off. Swallow mouthfuls of curry or of warm chocolate, of figs and asparagus and imagine them going straight to your nipples and clitoris, or to your penis. Just visualize the warmth, taste, shape and feel affecting you, making you swollen and hot, ready for love. Eat sparingly and slowly so you don't get overfull and bloated. Having strenuous sex on a full stomach isn't a recipe for love. This game is best played with tiny treats, luxurious nibbles and tasty titbits. Graze your way through a sumptuous spread, but make sure you actually eat small amounts over a period of time. Taste and devour a bit of everything and share small mouthfuls with your partner, to make the point and get the idea. Revel in contrasts. You can switch from hot to cold by taking a mouthful of ice or ice cream and then tonguing or sucking a part of your partner's body – earlobe or nipple, penis or clitoris. Having chilled and stimulated them, take a mouthful of something warm and repeat the exercise. Go from something crunchy and fresh to something sloppy and rich and see how the contrasting texture relates to your partner's body. The beauty of this game is that it is very flexible. You can surround yourself with the entire contents of a supermarket trolley. Or you can do it with just a take-away and a can of lager or a tub of ice cream. If you really want to go to town, you can put down a rubber sheet and pour your food all over each other and eat it off your partner's body. Some couples get a great kick from sploshy, messy sex where they dribble custard, cream and anything else squishy over each other and lick it off. Try it and see.

EAT ME

Few of us can resist the charms of our favourite foodstuffs, and you can harness your appetite for food to enliven another – your appetite for each other. Pat and Moira were both food lovers and their first date had been over a meal. But they'd never quite made the connection between food and sex until they saw a video of the film *Tom Jones*, which contains a scene where two potential lovers seduce each other over a table of food. Pat came home one night to find Moira waiting for him in the hallway. "Now, don't you give me no argument," she said. "I want you to go upstairs, have a shower and change into what I've laid out on the bed for you. Trust me, you'll be glad if you do! When you're ready, come down to the living room." Pat walked in to a scene of Eastern Promise. He balked at first. He said it felt silly, he was on a diet and was worried that the neighbours might call round. Moira smiled and kept good humoured through all his complaints and just fed him a prawn. Pat left the room and Moira just kept on nibbling. He eventually came back and had a glass of wine. And then a handful of peanuts. And then a spoonful of chocolate mousse, which he dribbled down Moira's cleavage. They spent three hours eating the feast, gradually working up to consuming each other.

Dribble spoonfuls of wine, cream or ice cream on each other and lick it off.

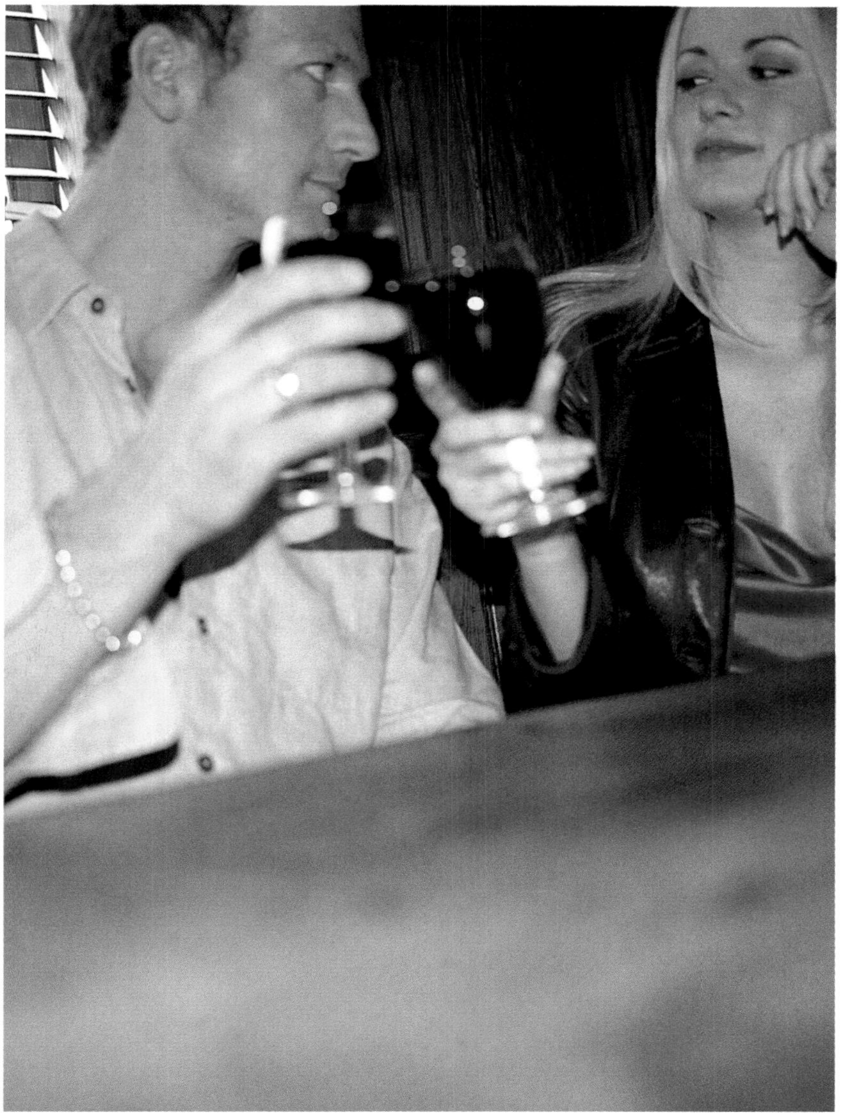

Recapture the thrill of your first date by meeting as strangers

FANCY MEETING YOU HERE

Having the same old sex with the same old partner can be at the root of a lot of dissatisfaction in relationships. Couples often use fantasy to put the excitement of a new relationship back into a settled one. When you're living together in a permanent relationship, making special time for you to be alone as a couple can often go by the board. Relationships can also very easily get into a rut. Once upon a time, when you were in your early days together, your sex lives were all adventure. Every encounter was thrilling, as you discovered new things about each other and yourselves. You knew what it was about each other that could set your pulse racing. Months or years on, it's all a bit stale and you might have mislaid that excitement. You'll hardly ever go out and when you do, it will be to do the same old things, in the same old fashion. You might be tempted to recapture the heady delight of a fresh encounter by flirting with a friend, neighbour, work-mate or even a stranger and possibly of having an affair. Sexual fantasy games can allow you to experience all this in safety, with your own lover.

If you want to put back the thrill of the new, consider playing the game of meeting and picking each other up, as strangers. Set the scene by arranging a table in the kitchen or living room to resemble a bar or café. Dress in outdoor clothes – put on a coat if it's winter, but leave something off underneath. If it's summer, don't wear any underwear. If it's winter, don't wear anything but your underwear, and make sure it's your briefest and sexiest. He should be carrying a newspaper. Set your mind to being new people. You're both single, your own and simply enjoying a quiet moment in a busy life.

Start the action with one of you sitting down and having a cup of coffee or a drink at the café or bar table. Of course, if you really want to go the whole hog, play this for real. Make a date to meet up somewhere new, where you aren't known. Pretend you don't know each other. Whether you're at home play-acting the entire thing or out, just play-acting the fact that you're strangers, once one of you is settled the other should come up and ask to share the table. Take a few moments to give each other a "once over" secretly. Do you like what you see? What do you find attractive? What particular part of that person's body would you like to touch? What would you like to do to and with them? When you've looked your fill, strike up a conversation: "Do you come here often? What do you do with your free time? Do you have a partner or are you available?" Let the conversation become more intimate: "What sort of person do you find yourself falling for? What sort of sex do you like?" As the chat gets hotter, she can let her coat fall open to show she is just in her underwear, or pull her skirt up to show she isn't wearing any. He can casually remark he's wearing a thong. Under the table and the cover of coats or a newspaper, both should let a hand sneak out to touch, fondle and explore the other's body. You can go as far as you like if the "café" is a pretence. How far you go if you're in a real bar is up to you, the lighting and the bar's other customers! Doing this for real can give you extra kicks, but do be careful. Don't do anything intimate when or where you could be seen or discovered and cause offence or discomfort to anyone else. It's bad manners for one thing. It's also illegal and can get you in considerable trouble. The best compromise is to pick each other up in public but continue any other activities once you get to somewhere private.

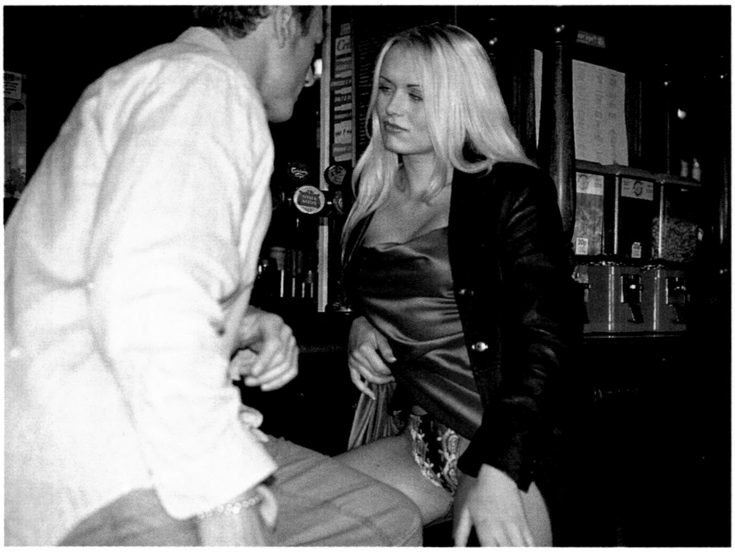

Two 'strangers' on to a sure thing

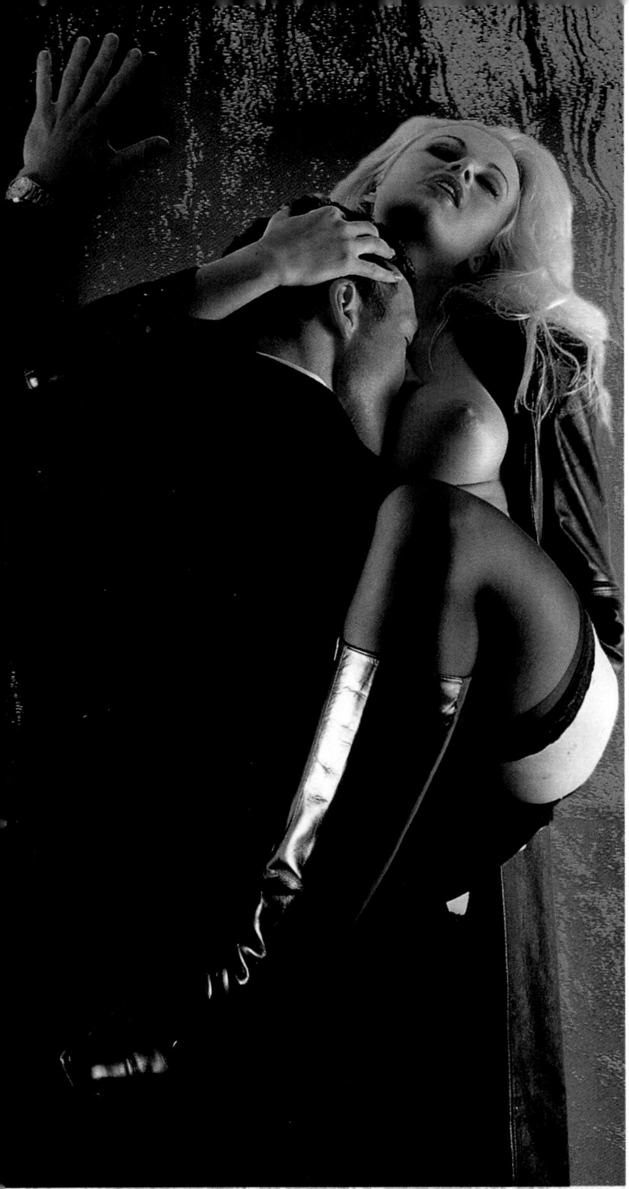

There are times when "wham-bam-thank-you-Sam" sex, fast and furious spur-of-the-moment sex, is what you need.

STRANGER IN THE NIGHT

Ali and Meera had been going out for three years and had settled into a comfortable routine. They never went out as a couple, but stayed in or occasionally met friends at their local bar. So Ali suggested they tried this fantasy game. They made a date to meet at a new café, in a week's time. Both went from work, so they had the added fear that the other would back out at the last moment. Both turned up, and neither recognized each other at first – Meera even tried to dissuade Ali from sitting with her for a few minutes until she realized it was him. She had bought herself a whole new outfit to wear and done her hair a different way. He had finally shaved off the moustache he'd had for months, and which she'd hated. They struck up a conversation. The discipline of having to make new introductions meant they talked about the things that interested them, as they hadn't done for ages. Meera had forgotten how much Ali liked wildlife programmes. Ali had forgotten how interested Meera was in travel, and how interesting she was when she got going about her main passion, French food. The excitement was increased by the near certainty that each was on to a winner. Both were astounded to find themselves falling in love with the other all over again – and getting a real sexual kick out of picking each other up. Now, they have a date once a month to meet a "new lover" in a restaurant, café or bar, and bring home all sorts of sexual tricks discovered on these evenings out to try at home.

FAMOUS FACES

Of course, we don't always confine our sexual daydreams to our own bedroom companions. A common fantasy involves having sex with someone we've known or seen. We might fantasize about being in bed once again with a past partner, but without the faults that probably ended the relationship. Or we might dream about a neighbour, colleague or simply someone we glimpsed at the bus stop. Probably the most common fantasy of this type is making love to someone famous. Sex with a celebrity is popular partly because you may have seen them in films or videos doing something that makes it easy to imagine having sex with them. The scenario, the characters and story has already been written for you. All you've got to do is to slot yourself into a scene that you have watched. Partly it's because the impression you may have got through the media is that they are very sexually experienced and would know what to do, so you can then imagine that sex with them would be very exciting and satisfying. But the other reason is that if, in your fantasy, someone with this status wants to make love to you, you must be very special.

Next time you make love to your partner, imagine it's really Brad or Julia, Leonardo or Catherine, Pierce or Cameron, Nicole or Tom who is in bed with you. Picture them the way you have seen them on the screen and put yourself in their co-star's place. If you think your partner has the self-confidence to cope with being ousted by the image of another – and you're prepared to accept the same – discuss this and see if you can say the names out loud. Madeleine had just such an understanding husband. She had had a thing for Sean Connery for years, and was rocked back on her heels one night when he spoke to her in the actor's unmistakable Scottish accent. He told her later he'd been practising for ages, and that he'd be perfectly happy if she sometimes called him Sean or James – "Bond, James Bond" – in bed. From then on, every so often they'd act out this fantasy and it always gave both Madeleine and her husband guaranteed sexual satisfaction.

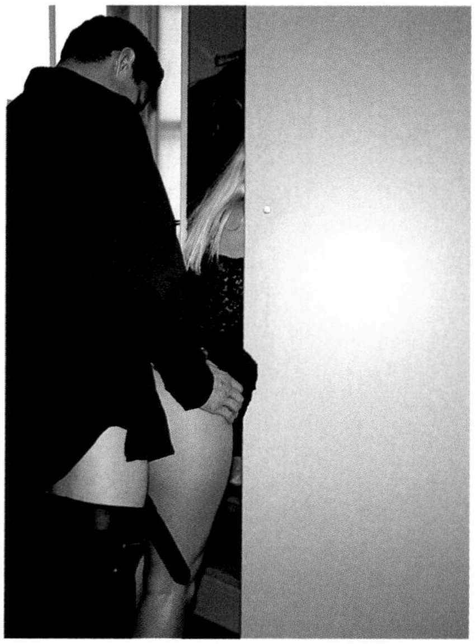

Fantasy sex – it's all in the mind

FACELESS LOVER

Another common way of improving the sexual experience is to imagine having sex with a stranger. Some people imagine making love with a person whose face they never see. With others the face and body is clear in their minds but is somebody they will never meet again. Sex in these circumstances is totally uncommitted – sex with no explanation, no price to pay and no consequences. Tara, for instance, had the fantasy of being in the ladies' in a restaurant when a man suddenly came in behind her. The lights were dim so she couldn't see his face, and when he sidled up and started kissing her neck and then swung her round to kiss her lips, long and passionately, it was too late to get a proper look at him. In her fantasy, they hear someone coming so she pulls him into a cubicle where they make love standing up, all the time hearing people coming and going outside. When they finally finish, he kisses her long and hard and then slips away, leaving her to tidy herself up before returning to her table and the unsuspecting friends she had left. Tara has told her boyfriend about her fantasy, which he thinks is "totally cool". Every time he takes her out for a meal, or she meets her girlfriends for a lunch or girls night out, he says, "Don't forget to go to the loo," and follows up with a whispered request for "one of those nights" – meaning a fantasy night when she gets home.

SPEEDY GONZALES

The fantasy of having sex with a stranger also keys into another popular sexual fantasy, that of quickie sex. Many men and women say the daydream of meeting someone whose face they don't even see, but with whom they share a sudden and burning embrace and hurried sex before going their separate ways again, is exciting because it is "no strings" sex. There's no foreplay, where you try to court and please your partner and make sure they're in the mood for love. If you compare leisurely, loving sex to a four-course banquet, which takes preparation, forethought, time and effort, sex with a stranger is the equivalent of the fast-food hamburger. You take it on the run, scoff it down and dash. It's the ultimate "I'm pleasing myself and you can do for yourself, too" sex, and can be amazingly exciting for that reason. So, too, is quickie sex. Having slow, considered, loving sex with full foreplay and a long afterglow can be both sexually satisfying and a great way of showing your feelings for your partner. But there are times when a "Wham-bam-thank-you-Sam" fits the bill even better. Fast and furious spur-of-the-moment sex has just as much of a loving message to pass to your partner. It tells them you're so overcome with passion that you must, simply MUST, have them there and then. It tells them that your feelings for them are so strong that you are prepared to risk anything to slake your immediate thirst for their body. And quickie sex, while being a bit of a cheat if that's the only sort you have, can be intensely arousing in certain circumstances. You'll be sure to find that the rush of adrenaline that the fear of discovery or interruption – and your insistence that you can't wait provokes – will aid arousal and orgasm. Quickie sex is also another way to return to first base. It's in the first few months of a relationship that we experience our fiercest, most intense feelings. That goes for the emotional link between us, as the pangs of love are at their strongest, but it's also noticeable in bed.

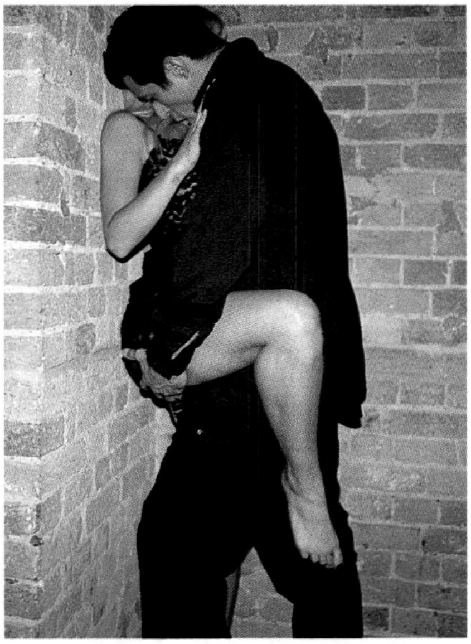

Quickie sex can sometimes fit the bill

It's the ultimate "I'm pleasing myself and you can do for yourself, too" sex, and it can be amazingly exciting.

Our sexual responses are probably at their most extreme at this time. When our relationship becomes more settled and stable, and probably more loving, the downside is that everything seems to be a bit short-lived and colourless. Quickie sex puts you back in the frame. You're doing it passionately, suddenly and spontaneously. You are likely to find yourself breathless again, and not just because you're in a hurry but because your partner and your feelings for them take your breath away once more.

TAKE YOUR TIME – NOT

Set yourself up by making sure you're in "quick release" clothes – something you can push aside to give you easy access for sex, but that you don't have to remove. A body stocking is a no-no, a thong, French knickers or nothing at all is fine. You can agree in advance what you plan, or one of you can surprise the other. Pick your moment; just before you know friends or relatives are due to knock on the door adds an extra tingle. Or you could catch your partner while you're out, walking in the country or seaside, in a bar, art gallery or carpark. Suddenly sidle up to or grab your partner and whisper in their ear that if you don't have sex with them that very moment, you'll explode. Kiss them, passionately and hungrily. Push your partner up against a convenient wall or seat, and undo zips and buttons. Pull clothes up, down and aside just enough to allow you to connect. With one eye peeled to make sure that you won't be caught out, take your partner and have fast and furious sex. Once you are finished, pull yourself together and resume whatever it was you were doing before. Carrying on as normal afterward is half the point of a quickie. Instead of lying in each others arms, basking in the afterglow, you smugly hug to yourselves the knowledge of what you've just, secretly and daringly, done. Use a condom and have some wet wipes on hand. That way there's no mess or leakage and after sex you can go straight on with whatever you were doing. As far as anyone else is concerned, nothing has happened. Apart from the silly grins on your faces, that is!

Haroon and Becky had been living together for a year when Becky started to feel their sex could do with a bit of a shake up. Haroon was a considerate lover and they usually had long, slow and very romantic sex. But the first time they had ever made it together was after a party, on a railway station on the way to Becky's home. It had taken all of two minutes and she still remembered every second. So Becky decided to surprise Haroon. One night, on the way back to their shared apartment, she insisted on going out of their way and changing trains at that station. She led him to the same spot – at the end of a platform, behind a pillar, and said, "Remember what happened here?" He did. "Want to do it again?" He did! They haven't stopped having leisurely sex, but every now and then they will throw in a quick one, to keep the juices flowing and the interest high.

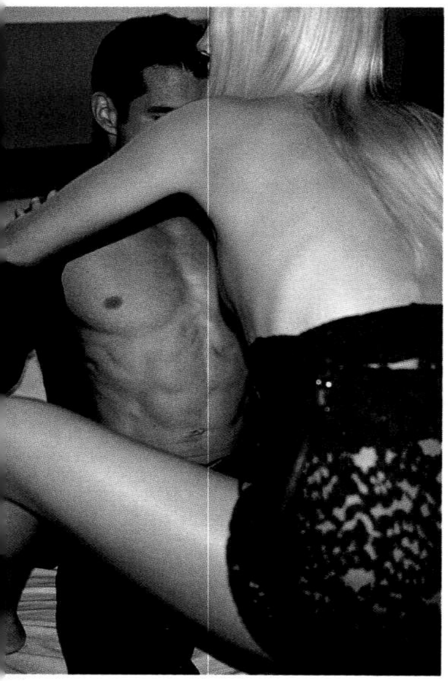

Two minutes of bliss

A BIT OF ROUGH

Imagining having sex using a certain amount of brutality or force to get our own way is probably one of the most common fantasies. Power and sex are inextricably entwined. They do say that power is the best aphrodisiac – it must be, because otherwise how could you explain the apparently irresistible charm of some of the world's richest but ugliest men? When we have difficulties in our own love lives, often it's because we feel powerless. We don't feel able to say what we want or be in control, of either our own needs or what happens between ourselves and a partner. Setting up a situation where you agree one of you is absolutely in control can be a great liberator. It makes the one in charge feel competent and strong. It's can also be quite a relief to the other one. You may only feel bad about not having a say when you think you should be making choices. When you agree to be told and led, you can relax and not worry, handing the reins over to the other person. That's also the reason why it works particularly well when you reverse the normal order of things, letting the one who's usually in charge in your relationship take a back seat and handing control to the one who is usually looked after.

Some people imagine using objects, materials and clothing to spice up their sex lives. High-heeled shoes, rubber or fur are all things that can add excitement. Lots of people also imagine sex which involves a certain amount of pain. There is a thin division between what gives us pain and what gives us pleasure. While you might not actually want to

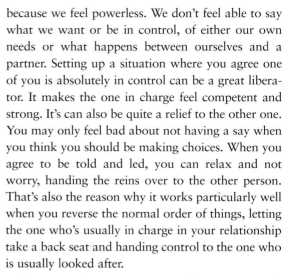

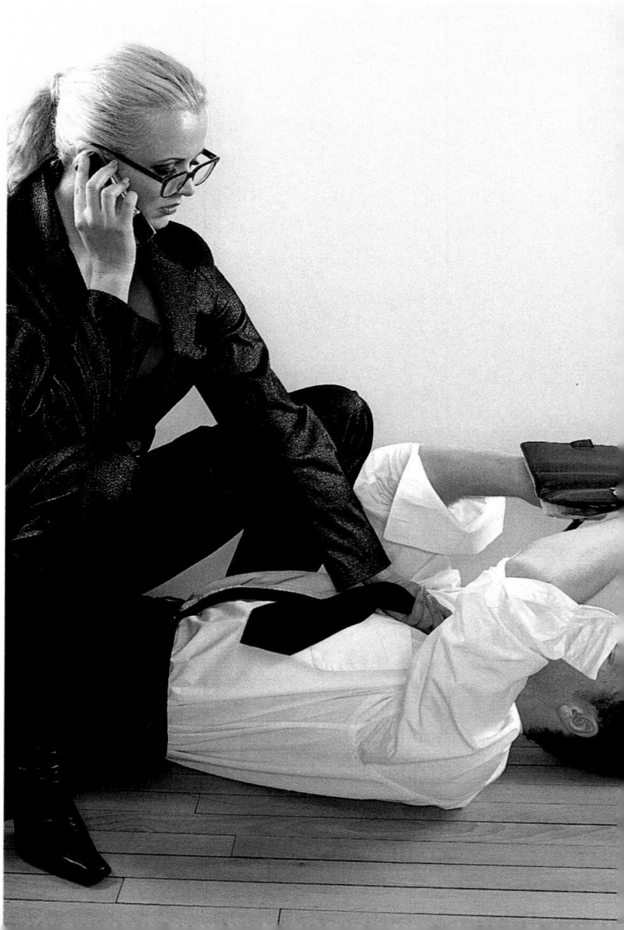

Right: Who's boss when you get home?

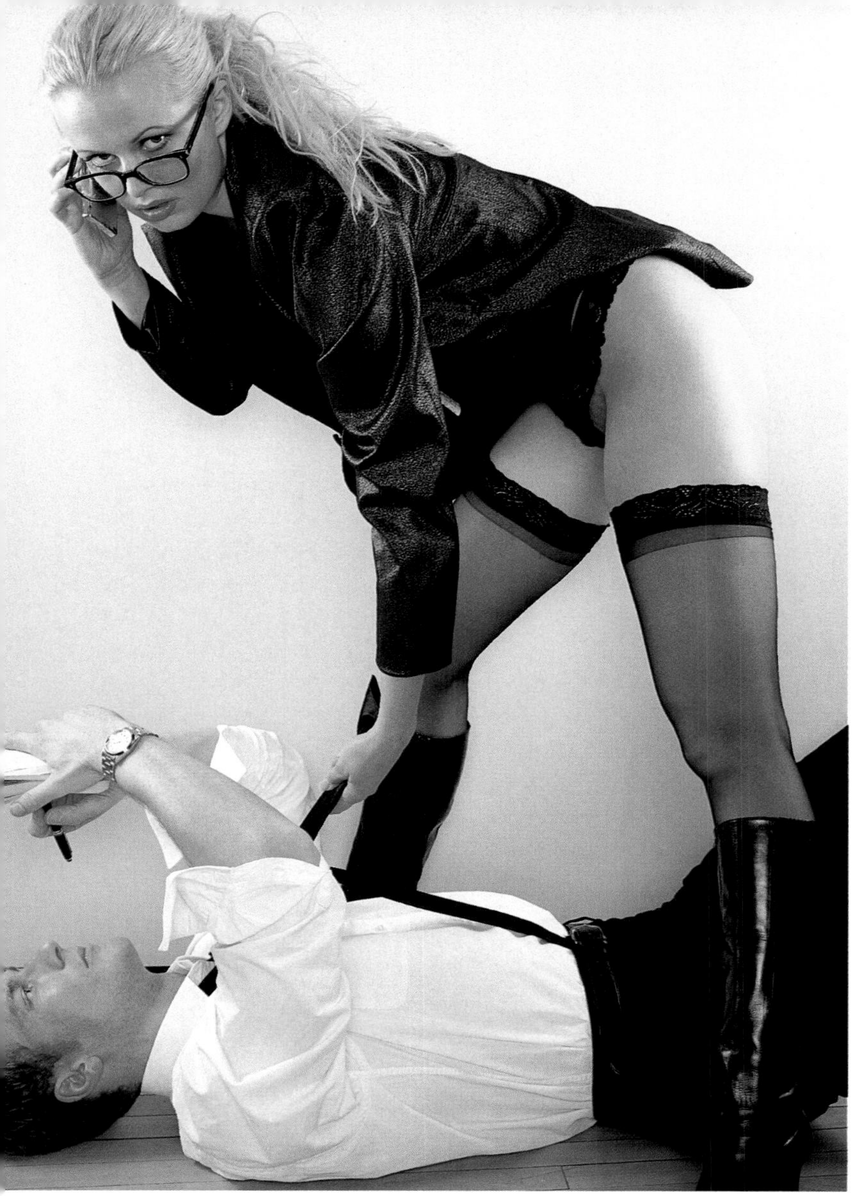

A powerful boss with high standards

DO WHAT THE BOSS SAYS

Set the scene by arranging a corner of a room like an office, with a desk and chair, a desk lamp if you have one, papers and pens. Dress in "business" clothes – a suit for him or dark trousers and a shirt and tie, sober skirt and blouse for her. But underneath, she should be wearing stockings rather than tights, and a sexy bra. Make sure you have a sash, tie, strap or a belt to hand or as part of your costume – you're going to need it. Imagine you're at the end of a busy day. You've a deadline coming up and an important project that has to be completed or the company is in trouble. She's the boss, a powerful lady who has high standards and never lets a mistake go by without soundly reprimanding the person who made it. He's her assistant, in awe of her, and he's made an error. He's been sitting there, nervous and on edge, hoping against hope she'll not have noticed it or will have decided to correct it herself, for speed. Some hope!

inflict pain, or have it inflicted upon you, while making love, you may find it exciting to imagine it happening. This can also be a way of working through any guilt about enjoying sex at all. If you think your desires are wrong or naughty, you may imagine being whipped or spanked as a way of being punished. In chapter 5 we looked at the world of the sub/dom and master/ slave scenarios. There are other, slightly less extreme versions of this, that do, however, have just as much an emotional punch to them. One is where you imagine one of you as the boss, the other the subordinate in a pretty excessive version of *Nine To Five*.

Power and sex are inextricably entwind. They do say that power is the best aphrodisiac.

Start the action by having him sitting at his desk. She should then come in and throw a sheaf of papers over him. Alternatively, if you have a mobile phone, she could ring him at his desk and order him into her inner sanctum. Or, she could set this up by ringing him earlier in the day, at his real place of work, to make an appointment, to tell him exactly what time he should go in to see her. Once there, she shouts the ceiling down. She's furious, and she's going to make sure he knows exactly how annoyed she is, and make him pay for putting her out. You could agree your own dialogue earlier, or use this: "For heaven's sake, look at this work. It's a mess. What did you think you were doing? I've a good mind to get rid of you." "Look, I'm really sorry. I'm sure I can fix it, just give me some time." He should plead, abjectly, for her understanding and forgiveness, but she remains unmoved and isn't going to forgive easily. "We don't have the time, you idiot. You're such an incompetent fool that I've done it myself. In fact, the job's finished and done with thanks to me and no thanks to you. So now everyone else has gone home and if you don't want the sack, you'll have to take your punishment." She strips off his tie and, using that and the sash of her dress, ties him to his chair. Hiking up her skirt to show her stocking tops, she then puts a hand down his trousers and brings him to attention. What happens next between them is designed to underline just how much in control she is, and how powerless and under her thumb he has become. With one hand stroking him and the other exposing her breasts to tease him, she laughs at him. "I bet you'd like to have a taste of these, wouldn't you? But you're far too incompetent to know what to do, you'll just have to let me show you how to do it!" He can beg for release and for the chance to show how good he can be, but she just keeps on teasing him. She unzips his trousers, slips off her pants and mounts him, all the while telling him that if he doesn't do a better job of staying erect than he did of the paperwork, he'll really be sorry. The boss may agree to untie him, but only so she can order her underling to go on his knees to kiss her feet, to perform oral sex or to grovel for her attention. He has to obey, because she's in charge. If she's in charge, she can keep him on the verge of climax and prevent him from actually coming for a surprisingly long time. The trick is to use the "squeeze technique". Take his penis in your hand, with your fingers along the top of the shaft, close to his body. Put the flat of your thumb just under the head of the penis – the glans – where the bridge of skin joins the bulbous head to the shaft. As he approaches the urgent point of no return, press firmly but gently with your thumb. You'll find he goes off the boil. The urge to come will recede and he will go a little soft, but will keep his erection. You can go on stimulating him until he reaches the same point, when you can repeat this – as many times as both of you can stand it.

Take his penis in your hand, with your fingers along the top of the shaft, close to his body.

LYING BACK AND TAKING IT LIKE A MAN

Plenty of men find being bossed around a real turn-on. Bob is one of them. Bob was a bit of a control freak. He was the sort of man who always had to keep the TV remote control on his side of the sofa. When he and his partner Linda went out for the night, Bob had to drive, even if they used her car. No one could ever tell Bob how to do anything – he knew best. Linda, who was a powerful business lady in her own right, had got used to letting Bob have his own way at home since it made for a quiet life. When he started getting sexual problems, finding it hard to get an erection and even more difficult to keep one, asking for advice was probably the hardest thing Bob had ever done. So he was gobsmacked when his therapist suggested it might help if he give up mastery for a change. But what emerged from talking it through was that Bob, like many men, suffered from command fatigue. It's hard work, always being the one to be in the lead. Having to risk rejection, having to make the first move, having to "be a man" by always being up for it, is tiring. So Linda and Bob agreed to try playing power games in this way. It was up to Linda to decide when, so Bob had almost forgotten it until one night, when she stormed into the living room and threw a bunch of papers all over him and dressed him down before undressing him. When he tried to get up, she pushed him down, and when he tried to tell her that he was tired, she rode over his objections – and was soon riding over him. To his amazement, Bob discovered his penis was up and hard before he knew what was happening, and it stayed hard until both of them had got what they wanted. Bob continued to be a power in his working life, but both of them found that they benefited from sharing control at home more equably.

TAKE THE PAIN

Fantasies can also allow you to experience a bit of rough or more but without the real pain. In this area, rape fantasies are quite common for both men and women, but don't get the idea that this means that either sex would really welcome actual force. Real rape and a rape fantasy have one enormous difference; in the first the raped person has no control at all over the scenario and no choice. In a fantasy, it is a scenario in your mind where you are actually in control. Then you can imagine yourself experiencing all sorts of sexual pleasures that guilt and embarrassment prevent you enjoying in real life. Imaging yourself being "forced" to do certain things is a sure-fire way of passing off responsibility for your sexual desires. But don't ever think that because anyone enjoys the idea that they'd accept the reality.

Claudine and Chris found a rape fantasy perked up their love life considerably. Claudine was a bit more sexually experienced than Chris, mainly because he came from a family with strict ideas about sex, which had left him with lingering guilt. He longed to be as relaxed as Claudine but found it hard. One night, he told her he'd had a dream where she had hit him and thrown him on the bed, taking him roughly and forcing him to have sex. What had surprised him was that, in spite of feeling real fear, he had been tremendously aroused. A week later, in the middle of a not-very-serious argument, Claudine suddenly grabbed Chris and wrestled him to the living room floor and literally ripped his jeans open. He was stunned – and even more stunned to find himself erect and ready in an instant. Since then, they have found that whether they talk about a scenario or play-act it, either provokes great sex.

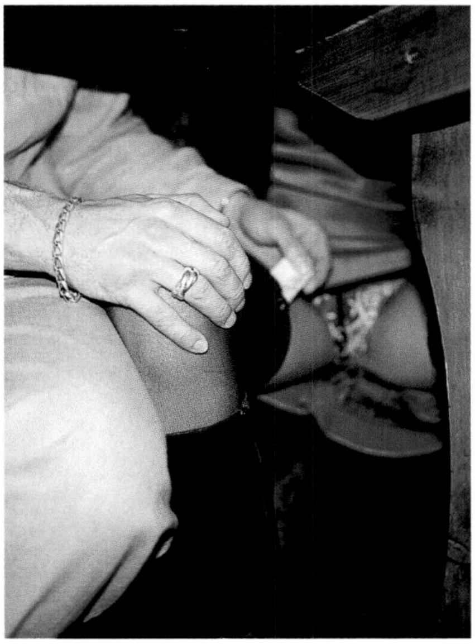

'Sex money' says you're worth it

THE POWER OF "SEX MONEY"

Paying for it is another reasonably common theme. Again, it's probably another way of removing constraints that would apply in real life. Pretending one of you is paying for sex has particular benefits for both payer and payee. Neither of you has to feel guilty for what happens. If you imagine being paid, you can feel an enormous sense of confidence and self-worth with someone thinking you are attractive enough or good enough to give money for it. When you are paid, you can feel that this "sex money" confirms that you're special. Imagining that your "mark" is prepared to give you cash for the privilege of having sex with you says that you and what you're offering is so good that it deserves such recognition and reward. When you are the one doing the paying, there is a different advantage – the customer is always right. If you're buying it, you can be totally self-seeking. You don't have to think about the other person's needs or pleasures but can concentrate on satisfying yourself and yourself only. You can also specify exactly what it is you want, without having to be shy, embarrassed or unselfish. This is why so many men use prostitutes in real life – the fact that they can get what they want and not have to bother about wooing and courting or thinking about the other person's needs. The other reason is that paid sex is felt to be "dirty" sex. And, often, there's nothing quite as thrilling and stimulating as being very naughty indeed. It's like sloshing around making mud pies. There's plenty of fun in the sheer sensuality of feeling it squish between your fingers, but even more enjoyment to be had from the knowledge that mother has told you not to! Imagining you're involved in the business of buying and selling sex can make your encounter seem sleazy and bad. And while that's not a recipe for happy sex in real life, it can be a definite turn-on in fantasy time.

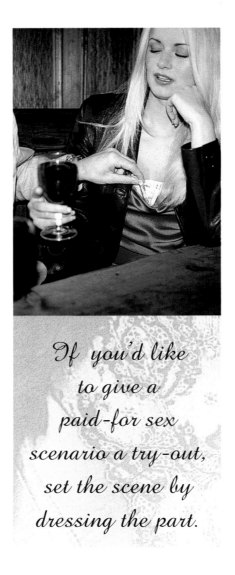

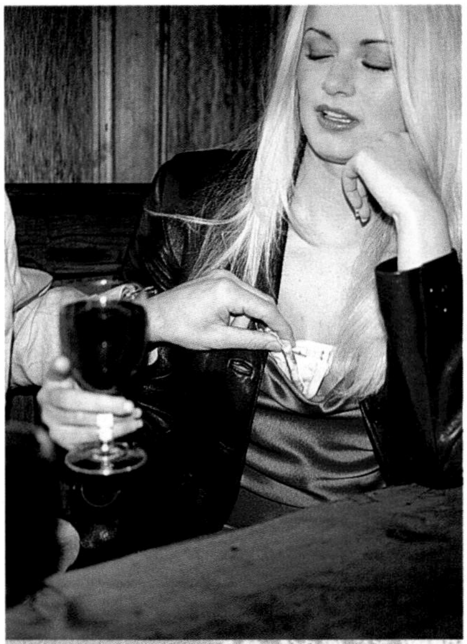

If you'd like to give a paid-for sex scenario a try-out, set the scene by dressing the part.

If you'd like to give a paid-for sex scenario a try-out, set the scene by dressing the part. The one who is to act the part of the sex worker should put on tight, revealing and cheap clothes. She can dress tartily in very short skirt or Lycra leggings and cropped top, with heavy make-up. If he's to be the rent boy, tight, ragged jeans or cut-offs, a T-shirt with cap sleeves or a shirt open to the waist will do. Torn jeans, by the way, is rent boy fashion. It says he does oral, because that's how his jeans come to be out at the knees. We tend to assume that all straight sex workers are women, and all clients are men. That isn't actually true, and it certainly shouldn't cramp your style. If she's going to get a kick out of being good enough to be paid to do it, so is he.

Both of you are likely to be a bit nervous. The sex worker is world-weary and cynical, having seen it all before. Nothing a client asks can shock or surprise. Start the action by having the buyer, feeling excited and determined to get what they want, approach the sex worker and ask, "Are you available?" "Depends. What are you looking for?" The buyer can then say exactly what they'd like. It might be a "quickie", for sex standing up, in an alley way; "a hand-job" for masturbation; "an oral" for oral sex; or "round the world" for everything – oral, anal and straight sex. You could specify that you want the sex worker to do all the work, making you come while you lie there being serviced, or you can insist that you want to take your pleasure from them as they stand or lie there, not moving. Or, you can ask that the sex be like making love – but they do have to touch and caress you as and when you tell them to. "That'll cost you," the sex worker can say, and they should then name a price. Alternatively, they may object to what's asked for and name another similar, but easier, sex act. The sex worker may also, for authenticity, demand that the client wears a condom and then be prepared to haggle if the client offers to pay double for sex without one. When they finally agree and the buyer hands over the cash, the sex worker leads the way up to the bedroom. Once the price is paid, the worker has to do what the customer says, as long as it is what they have asked and paid for. To put an extra edge to the negotiations, use real

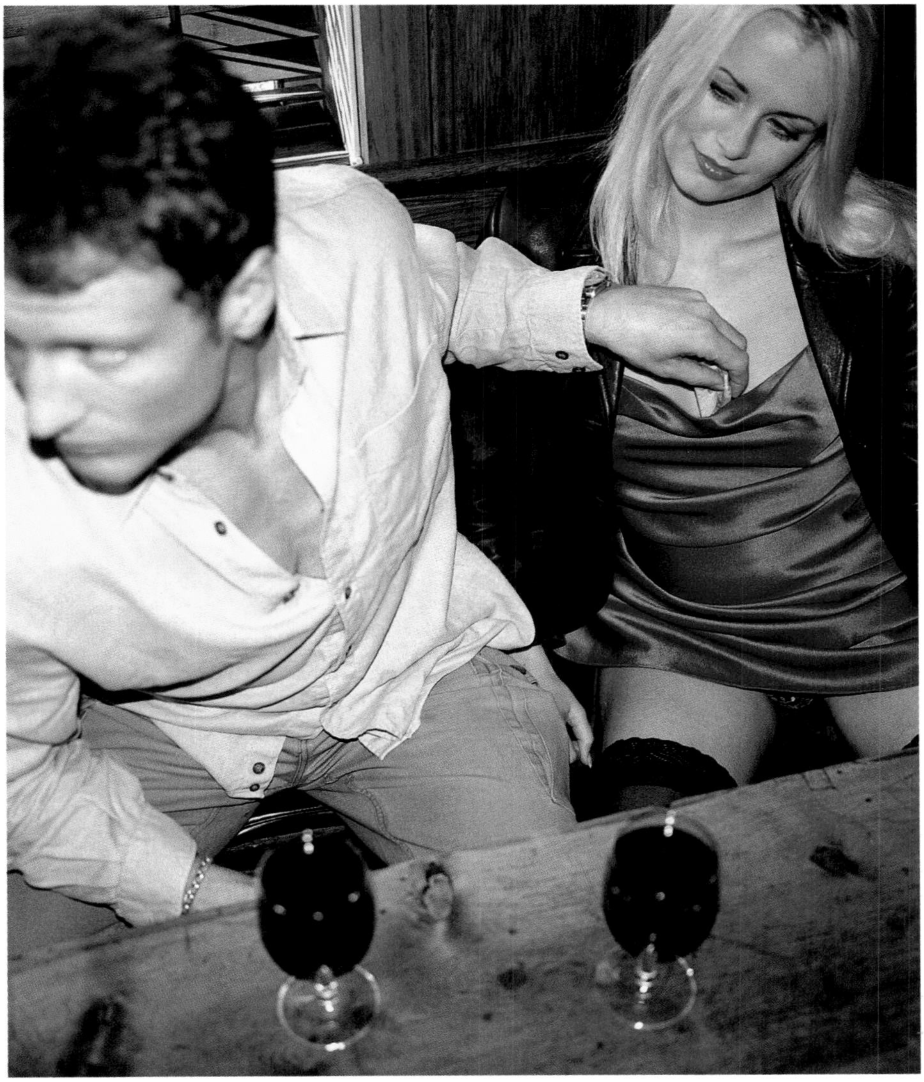

Bought and paid for, both can have guilt-free sex

money. The sex worker gets to keep the cash and buy themselves a treat with it.

BOUGHT AND PAID FOR

Danni had always wanted to try oral sex, and suspected her husband Craig had too. But both of them had family backgrounds in which sex was a taboo subject, never talked about out loud. She had a feeling that if he was given free rein, that was what he would ask for. So she suggested they played a game of forfeits, and when she won, she said they should try a paying-for-it game as an exercise. Craig was reluctant at first, and was only coaxed into it when Danni promised – "...cross my heart and hope to die" – that she meant it, he really could ask for his heart's desire and she wouldn't be shocked or critical. Emboldened by this, sure enough, he asked for oral sex. Danni would have blushed furiously and probably turned him down if he'd asked as Craig. Since he was an anonymous punter and she was a "working girl", she took it in her stride. Their first attempt wasn't the best blowjob in the world – neither cared – but both were well satisfied. They found they could talk about sex far more easily when they could do it as punter and pro, and it gradually meant they could be more open in real life, too.

NEWBIE TO LOVE

You can make the same attempt at seeing yourself as special by going to exactly the other extreme and imagining virgin sex. Making love to a virgin – someone who would give themselves to you as the sexually experienced one, for your guidance and expertise – can be a stroke to your self-esteem. The reverse scenario is equally popular and it can be an equal sexual charge to imagine being seduced by someone much older and more experienced who guides you and so takes the pressure off you to perform. This fantasy also gives you the boost to your ego that you have a quality that they, with all their experience, value. That's another fantasy that can make you feel special, if in real life you feel that no one appreciates you.

There's nothing quite as exciting as first-time sex. As a teenager, taking those original steps from holding hands, to tentative kissing through to petting, you would have been in an agony of uncertainty. The mixture of terror, curiosity and anticipation made your pulse race and your stomach churn and it would have added to your sexual arousal. All that adrenaline racing round your body would have joined with those teenage hormones to make first-time sex thrilling enough to have you coming almost as soon as you touch. There's still an enormous mystique attached to taking someone's virginity. Both men and women can be ecstatic at the thought that they might be their partner's first lover, the one who introduced them to the world of sex. Even if you've known your partner for years, you can recapture that kick by playing at being, or seducing, a virgin.

One of you is going to be an innocent. Whoever picks the chance to go first is the virgin, or you can toss a coin to decide which of you will be the seduced and which of you will be the seducer this time. The winner puts themselves in the shoes of a school pupil stirred by the first glimmerings of sexual curiosity and desire. Our virgin is a stranger, so far, to shared bliss but not a total newcomer to the sensual pleasures. He or she has discovered the delight of self-pleasuring and so is all the more ready to be initiated into the world of adult sex. They've fumbled around with someone their own age a few times, but that seemed clumsy and unexciting. They've had "crushes" on film and pop stars, and had quite a few sexual fantasies about them. Recently, our young virgin has been having even more explicit daydreams about a particular friend of a brother or sister. The other one of you will play this person, an Older Friend of a brother or sister. You're sexually experienced, confident and good-looking. You've met the young Virgin before, but never really noticed them. You're calling round to see your friend, with nothing on your mind.

Set the scene by arranging cans of soft drink, schoolbooks and a teenage magazine around the living room. Put some music on, or turn on the TV or radio to something a teenager would watch or listen – an Aussie soap, for instance. The Virgin should be dressed in school uniform – a plain skirt or trousers and a white blouse or shirt with a uniform-style tie.

THERE'S A FIRST TIME FOR EVERYTHING

Start the action by imagining Virgin has come home from school to find the house empty. They're just about to settle down to homework or a coffee or soft drink when the door bell rings and it's that friend of the brother or sister, calling round to see them. Virgin invites the Older Friend in for a coffee, feeling both tongue-tied and thrilled. The rest of the family won't be back for ages, so here's a chance to have this sophisticated company to themselves. As well as having set the scene and imagined the state of mind of both the participants, have a few lines of dialogue prepared. Start off with Virgin telling Older Friend, "They'll be back soon. Why don't you wait? I'll get you a coffee." Wherever friend sits, Virgin then tucks themselves in close, sharing a sofa or balanced on an armchair seat. Older Friend isn't exactly averse to being sociable, either. There may be an age gap, but it's very flattering when you realize that an attractive, nubile youngster is making eyes at you. So the Older Friend starts off being polite, asking about school studies and kindly enquiring what the young person hopes to do when they leave school. But then they pick up one of the magazines and realize that sex figures large in these. The teasing becomes more explicit: "So this is the sort of homework you do, is it? What about the practical, how much of that have you done?" Lifting the

There's nothing quite as exciting as first-time sex. As a teenager, taking those original steps from holding hands, to tentative kissing through to petting, you would have been in an agony of uncertainty.

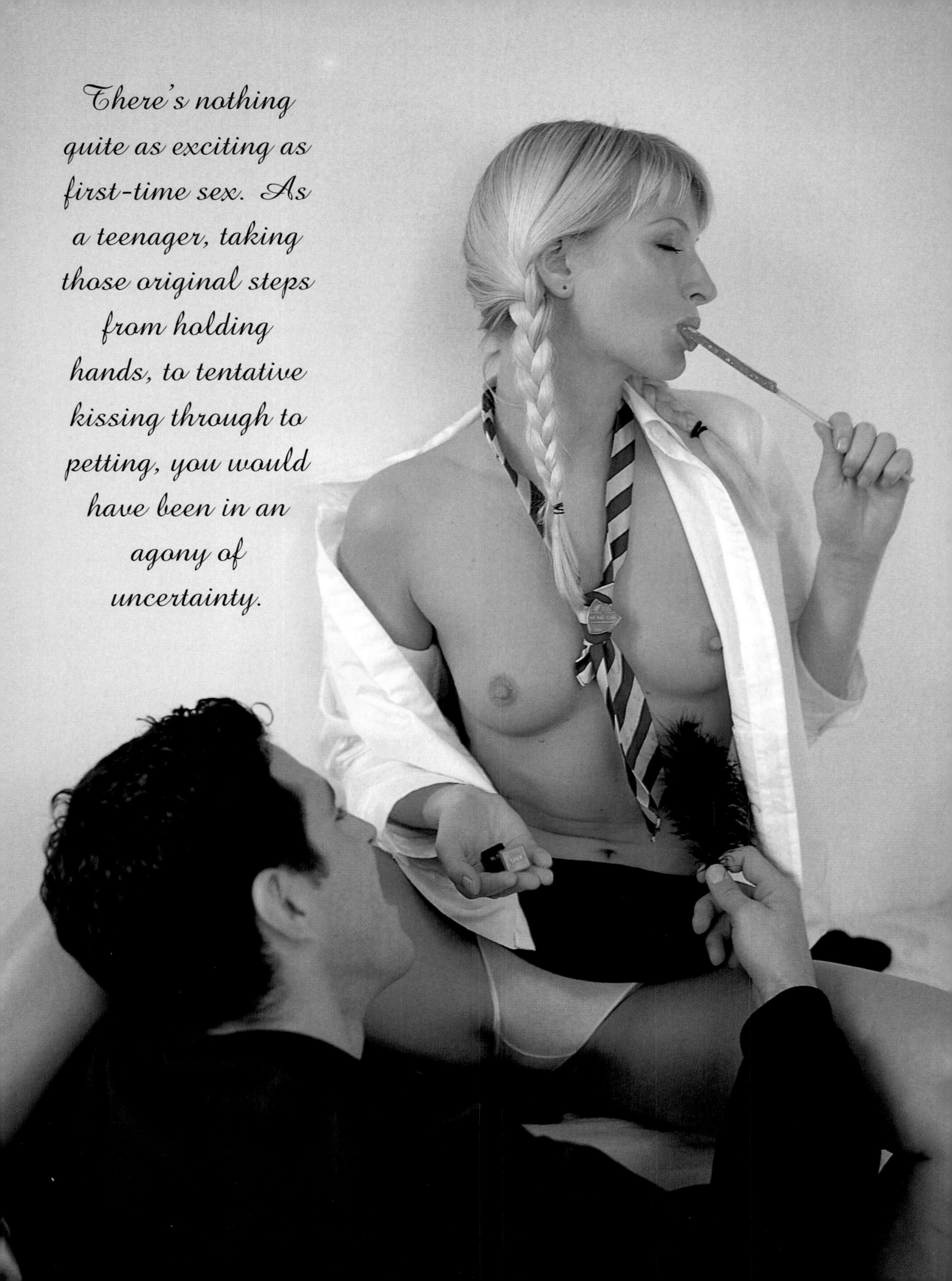

drink, Older Friend accidentally-on-purpose spills some on the uniform shirt. "Hey, I'm really sorry, I'm so clumsy. You'll have to take that off or it will stain and you'll get told off. Here, let me help you." Riding over any protests, Older Friend unbuttons the shirt and tugs it out of the waistband. They're face to face, up close and personal, and Older Friend leans in and takes a long, lingering kiss. "Well, here's your chance to get a few lessons ahead." Older Friend then offers to find the lesson for the day, and show Virgin how to do it.

Playing this game allows you to recall what first excited you about sex in general and your partner in particular. You might find yourself recollecting a particular sexual position, a particular sexual sound, a particular texture, article of clothing, scent or taste that lit you up the first time and still has the power to do it for you. You may not be able to bring it to mind just by thinking, remembering or reminiscing. Act it out and it may all come flooding back, to dramatic effect. This particular version of the scenario is only a suggestion. Think and talk about it, and it's probable that you and your partner may find a whole play in your own imagination, from your own memory, that you'd like to re-run or re-invent for your very own, private, virgin experience. Many people, for instance, had their first sexual experience in a car. If you have a garage or parking space that isn't overlooked, you could replay the end of the date that was your first time. And don't assume that he needs to be the Older Friend, she the Virgin. We tend to imagine, when a virgin is seduced by an expert, that it's a girl being won over by a man. One of the most potent myths, for both men and women, is of the older woman – a "Mrs Robinson" – taking a young lad in hand and leading him to manhood by teaching him some tricks. Add an extra boost to your love life by playing this one with her in charge.

BACK TO FIRST BASE

Playing "seduce the virgin" can have a dramatic effect on a sex life that has gone a bit stale and limp. Jan and Nick tried it because their love life had got into a rut after ten years of marriage. Sex was boring and unexciting, and they couldn't remember what it felt like to be excited by each other the way they used to be, every time. When it was suggested they go back to first principles and try this, they thought they'd collapse in giggles and not be able to carry out the scene. But both were surprised at how easy it was when they pretended they were putting on an act for the local amateur dramatics society. Both of them took some time to imagine what they would say to each other in the scenario, which they had talked about. Jan wrote out a few lines for both of them, but told Nick he could change his as he wanted, to surprise her. Once they got caught up in the action, they forgot they were supposed to be acting and played it for real. It brought back memories of their early days, with a twist. Jan played the Virgin and Nick the Older Friend. When they had first met, it was Jan who had been more sexually experienced. On the first night they had had sex, it had been Jan who took the lead. Nick had always felt a little embarrassed about that. Not only did they find the game brought a new charge to their sex life, it also allowed Jan and Nick to feel that they'd rewritten their original "first time", this time with him playing the experienced one. This gave him renewed self-confidence and made it special again for both of them. Having played Virgin Nights with Nick as the adult, they did it again with Jan as seducer. This time, Nick enjoyed it even more. He could allow himself to be led by the hand once he also felt he could take charge.

FACE IN THE CROWD

There are few people who won't have wondered at some time or other what it would be like to have three in a bed. A fantasy shared by many people is having sex with two or more people, with both or all of them being of the opposite sex, or with a mixed couple or a group. There is the kick of imagined numbers vying for your charms. The temptation to make love to, or be made love to by, more than just your own partner at a time comes from a wish to have your ego massaged as well as your body. The thought of having one or more people watching as we make love to a third, approving of us and admiring our moves, appeals to the exhibitionist in us. When you imagine someone of the same sex, you may be expressing a degree of competitiveness, or you may be saying

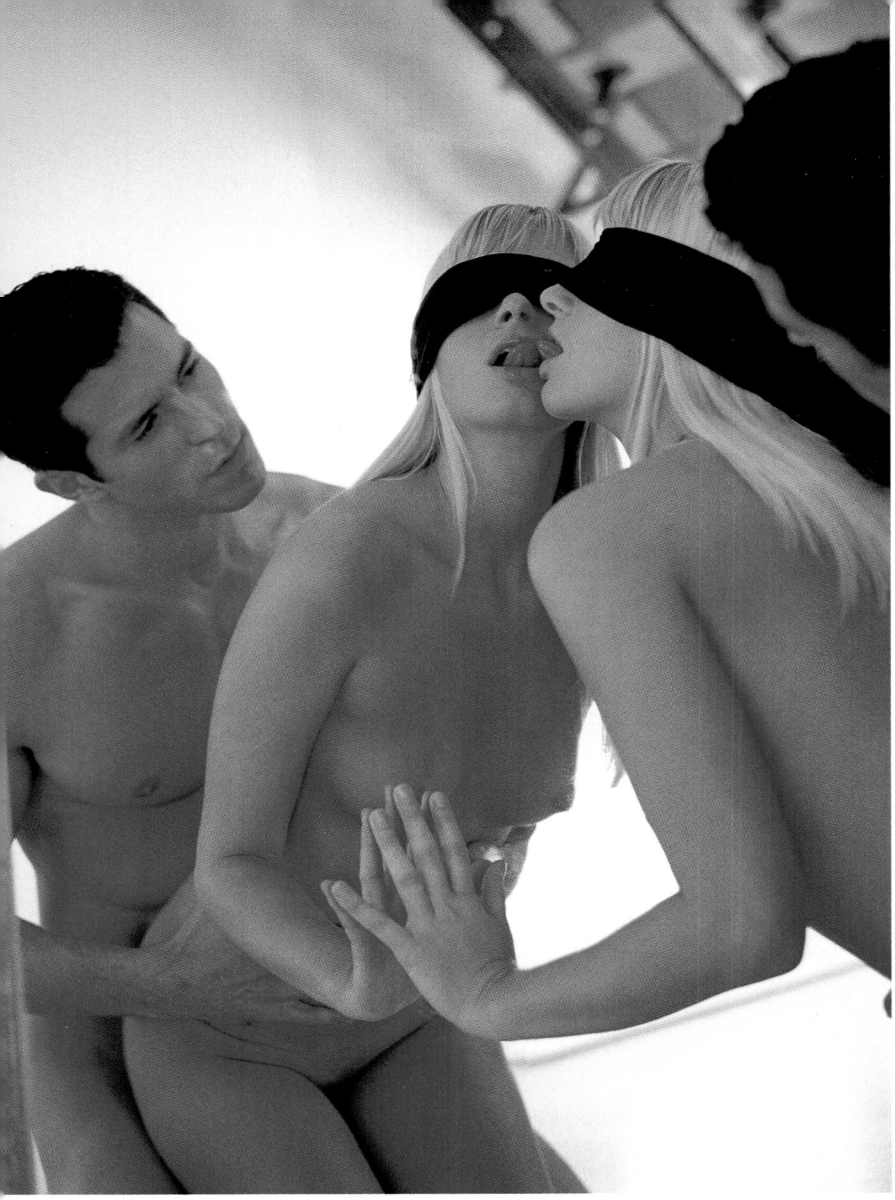

Using a mirror and fantasy you can have the thrill of group sex without the dangers

desires to be so large that you can be fulfilled only by a group and that you need two or more people to fill you or handle you. If you can cope with more than one lover, it suggests that your sexual abilities are extreme. Being spread around in this way means that you also don't have to worry about relating to one person. You are there for them to pleasure.

Whatever, thinking that there are extra bodies in the bed with you can really put a kick into the proceedings. Carrying it out for real, however, can cause problems. You've the worry of sexual infections. You've also the fear of competition and of emotional entanglements. The last thing you want to happen is for your partner to decide that someone else does it better for them, or for you to fall for a person other than your partner and have to deal with the fallout. Infidelity in fantasy is only that, a fantasy.

The thought of having one or more people watching as we make love to a third, approving of us and admiring our moves, appeals to the exhibitionist in us.

you would like a companion to back you up, someone to confirm that your sexual tastes are OK. If you are imagining yourself, however, with two or more people of the opposite sex, you may well be saying that you feel yourself and your In life, it's betrayal. Take it from me, this is one of those fantasies – and there are plenty – that are more attractive in the imagination than in reality. Playing at it, however, allows you to experience the thrill with none of the drawbacks.

Prepare the scene by placing one or more large mirrors around where you are going to make love – in the bedroom, bathroom or living room. You can place one upright against a wall and/or prop one up along the side of the bed, so that it will reflect you as you lie down. If you don't have any mirrors that will do, you can create the illusion of other people just by using the blindfold and suggestion. Turn the lights down low, perhaps illuminating the room with just candles or the light from a door left ajar. Have a blindfold, a scarf or a tie on hand as you go to your partner.

Start the action by putting on some music. Choose a smoochy, sexy number, and one that is not just instrumental. Make sure there are voices apart from your own to be heard. Then begin cosying up to your partner and saying, "You know we've been talking about those friends of ours who like to swing? Let's go upstairs, because I think they're planning to join us tonight." Blindfold your partner and lead them up to the dimly lit bedroom. Start seducing your partner, kissing, caressing and undressing them, pressed up against the mirror if you have one. When both of you are fully aroused ask, "Whose hands are these? Are they mine or are they John or Jane's? They're here." If you've a mirror, slide the blindfold off and allow your partner to see reflections in the half-light. If not, keep the blindfold fully or partly on. Keep up a running commentary about what the other people in the room are doing to your partner, and to each other and to you. "He's touching you on your breast. Now she's holding me. That's his hands between your legs. Can you hear her coming?" Use a vibrator, a feather or a silk glove to make sure both of you feel different textures and temperatures in the touches you are experiencing all over your bodies. If you really want to fool your partner's senses, consider this. Ever had someone sneak up behind you, cover your eyes and cry, "Guess who?" You can usually tell if it's your partner by their smell, whether you realize it or not. You know the soap, toothpaste and cologne they normally use. But you can also identify that subtle odour that is their own body smell, and which is highly sexy to your nose. This can make it hard to establish the illusion of it being someone else. To make you feel that it isn't only the two of you in the bedroom, splash the pillow beforehand with a perfume or aftershave that neither of you use.

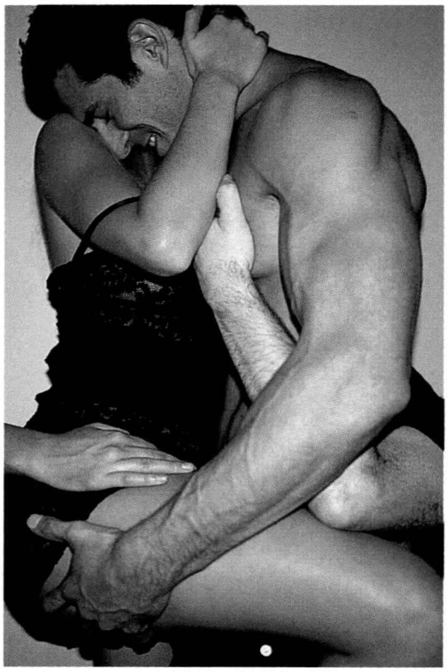

Three's a crowd except in a fantasy sex game

TOO GOOD FOR JUST ONE LOVER

Gary had always wanted to try three in a bed, ever since he had seen an adult video as a teenager that featured an orgy. But he was madly in love with his partner, Mandy, and not only was she uncertain about the idea, he also didn't want to share her with anyone else, male or female. She suggested that they have a go at it in fantasy. Gary was sceptical and couldn't see the point, but reluctantly agreed to go along with it. Mandy sprung it on him one night, after they had gone to bed and were lying in the dark. She told him some friends of hers were coming round and that she'd given them the key. She then spun a tale, describing hearing them come in downstairs, walking up the stairs and getting into bed with them. By that time, she and Gary were having sex and he didn't know which way was up! Next morning, he still wasn't totally sure it had been a fantasy, especially when he found a pair of men's underpants that he knew weren't his on the bedroom floor along with a thong he'd never seen Mandy wear. What both of them were sure of was that it had resulted in one of the best nights of sex they'd had so far. Both of them agreed that playing the game was as far as they'd want to go, but that the fantasy was a welcome addition to their sex life.

♦ WATCH THIS!

Add a few more bodies and you are in the land of orgy and here there is the added element of watching and being watched. Fantasies about watching other people making love or of taking part in sexual laboratory tests and having your sexual prowess measured, or of making love with an audience of applauding people, are very common for both men and women. The reason is probably because most of us feel a bit unsure of our skills in bed. We'd love to think that we're sexual experts, but most of us fear we're actually sexual inepts, which is why imagining you're the headline act in a sex show is a not only a popular sexual fantasy but a very reassuring one. If you want to try it, picture yourself in front of an eager, admiring and applauding audience. Suppose yourselves in demand to show them exactly how you do it. By imagining your fans urging you on to new heights as you demonstrate your skills in the arts of sex, you can give yourselves more than a thrill. It can also help you both to feel and be more confident in the way you please each other. As you think about people watching, envying and wanting to copy you, you can start accepting that perhaps what you're doing and the way you're doing it is worth some praise.

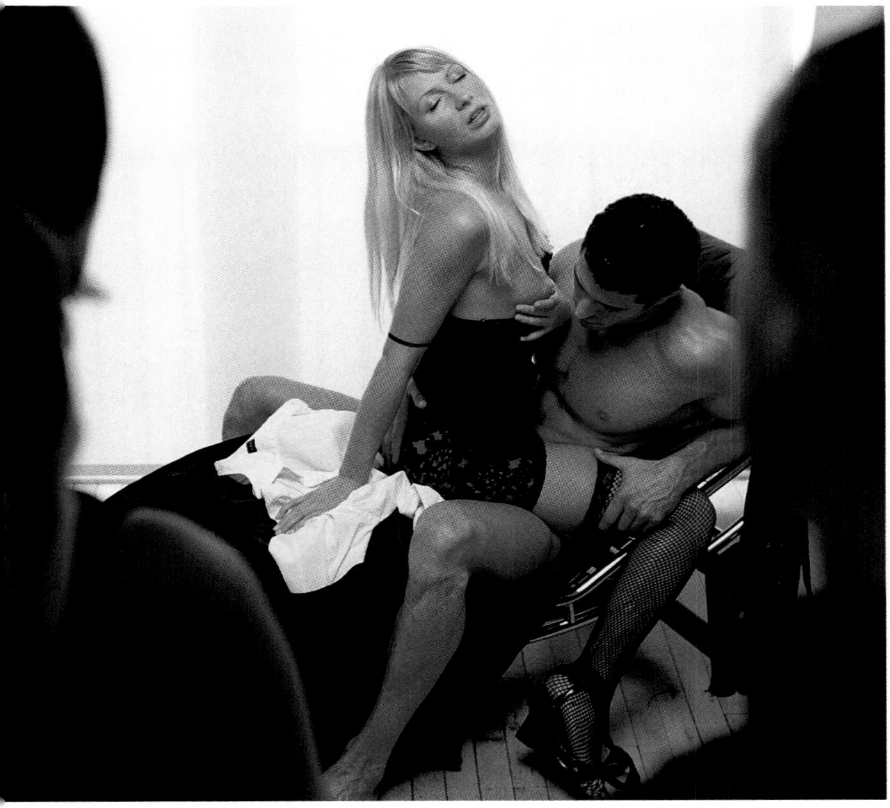

Putting on the performance of a lifetime

Arrange the scene by making a stage set in your bedroom or living room. You can use a rug to outline the limits of a small stage, or use your own bed as the set. Dim the lights, leaving one light, the spotlight, shining on the central area. Pick a soundtrack with a pounding beat and appropriate lyrics that get you going – make sure you have at least an hour of music to work to. Have a container of oil or cream within reach. Then prepare yourselves. Use glamour make-up to give yourselves a stage sparkle. Dust glitter make-up on breasts, backsides and genitals. Dress in thongs and clothes that you can shrug out of and remove easily. You'll both be feeling the butterflies any performer gets before a show, but also the quiet confidence of true professionals. You're so good at this, you know you're going to get a good reception and show your audience a thing or two.

As you hear the music coming up to your big number, start the action by both putting the final touches to your make-up and costumes and then make your entrance. Step into the spotlight, twirl each other round with a shimmy and a shake and get down to business. Strip each other of your clothes. Take your time about it – each article should come off slowly, with a tease and a flourish. When you're down to nothing, fetch the bottle of oil or cream from the side of the stage and slowly spread it all over each other. Arouse and excite each other and, to the imagined howls and screams of your frenzied audience, make love on the stage, in front of them all. Every move should be larger than life, played to the gallery. You can imagine your fans at the back of the room standing on the tables and urging you on, and your gestures should be large enough for them to be able to see exactly what you are doing to each other. After all, this is what they've paid to see. Afterward, don't forget to congratulate and praise each other, as real performers do. A few high-fives and "Nice moves!" will finish the act properly.

Of course, you can make up your own act. Boogie Nights and Disco Dancing aren't the only ways to perform a live sex act in front of an audience. Perhaps you'd like to imagine yourselves doing a Dracula, sweeping a cloak over your partner as you gnaw at their neck. Or being a Gladiator, knocking six bells out of each other in your Lycra and helmets before getting down on the mats. Or one of you can do a solo performance, pleasuring themselves for their audience of one. Or you can start the act with one of you in the audience, being invited up to strut your stuff with the professional performer. It's your script, so get writing! One tip is to make a recording of a stage show, one that has plenty of audience participation in the form of whoops, claps and shouted comments. Play it as you play this game and try to pace your performance to the audience reaction.

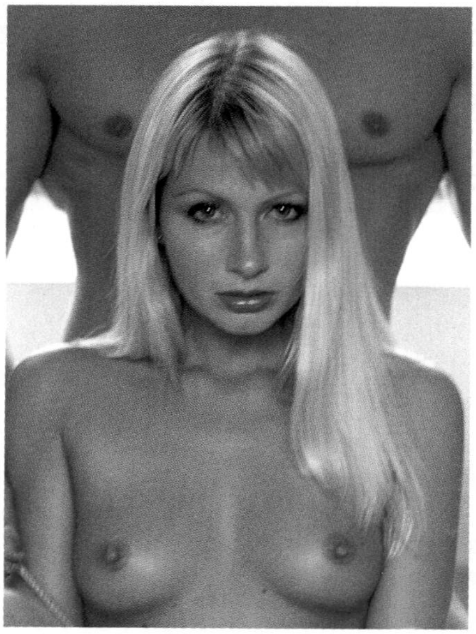

The only rule is "do no harm" to anyone else or yourself

HOW DID I DO?

One couple who really benefited from play acting a fantasy of performing in front of an audience were Mike and Tina. Mike was always a bit of a boaster and loudmouth when it came to tales of sexual prowess. When he was out with his friends, he'd make remarks and drop hints about how good he was. But his girlfriend Tina knew the truth, that he was actually convinced he was a poor lover. He was riveted by a television programme about the porn industry, and couldn't stop talking about one of the featured men, and how it must feel to be able to perform in public. One night, he'd tell her he could do that too. Another, he'd say he'd be terrified and so would any normal man, and not be able to get it up. So Tina started building him up, telling him he could do it if he tried. Knowing he'd probably refuse to co-operate if she asked him, she set up this fantasy game and sprang it on him one night. He came home to find the living room set up as a club, the music playing and Tina in a thong and basque, ready to go. Mike hesitated at first but then fell in with the game and loved it, performing like a hero. The sex was terrific, but the side effect was that he became far more self-confident and far less of a show-off and braggart. Now he felt he had something to brag about, he kept it between Tina and himself.

SAME GENDER SEX

Straight men and women often have fantasies about having sex with someone of their own gender. This can be exciting partly because we often think such sexual expression is forbidden and different. Partly it can be because you are actually imagining making love to yourself. It really doesn't mean that you would prefer to switch from having opposite-sex to same-sex partners. It's also worth noting that gay men and women also sometimes fantasize about having straight sex. Again, it doesn't mean they are thinking of changing orientation, which is not a matter of choice anyway. It all comes down to the fact that the spice of fantasies is that they allow you to experience and explore that which you might not like in real life.

Steph often found herself thinking about other women when she and her husband made love, but was frightened and ashamed of herself. Then her best friend, who she knew was in love with and faithful to her own husband, and was sure she was straight, confessed to similar dreams. Steph's friend just laughed about it and said it gave her own husband a sexual thrill to hear her imaginings. So Steph tentatively raised the matter with her husband, and was stunned to see him react with enthusiasm. She now often imagines herself making love with friends, film stars or pop singers and her man co-operates with a will by making "gay sex" nights occasions when they have long, slow, non-penetrative sex using a vibrator.

MAKE IT A REHEARSAL

Sexual fantasy can be used as a way of trying out certain sexual variations or acts to see if you might like them – rehearsals for a possible real thing. Oral sex is a great turn-on for many people but you or your partner may be put off by fears of an unpleasant taste or smell. In your imagination, your own or your partner's body can be "good enough to eat" and you can picture the deep satisfaction of sharing this very intimate sexual treat. Still common, but not quite as popular and moving toward the bottom of the top-twenty scale of fantasies, is imagined sex with animals or with a member of a different race. Sex with "the other", whether another species, another race or even – for "X Files" and "Star Trek" fans – some being from another planet, is sex freed from constraints and guilt. All races have fantasies about members of another race being somehow more uninhibited in sexual matters and therefore more exciting.

I hope that by now you are convinced that sexual fantasizing is normal, common, harmless and enjoyable. If, however, you find you resort to it constantly you might ask yourself if there are real problems in your life that you are trying to avoid or escape by fleeing deeper and deeper into reality. If fantasizing has become so essential that you can't have sex successfully without it then you should definitely look for help. That said, fantasy should be enjoyed as fun with the additional benefit that it costs nothing and needs nothing but yourself or a partner to use it. The cherry on the cake is that almost everyone is a fantasy figure to someone and it can be its own boost to fantasize about who might be fantasizing over you. It's also reassuring to recognize that the partners of all our accepted sex gods and goddesses, like film and pop stars, must also fantasize. It's nice to think that a Mr Julia Roberts or a Mrs Brad Pitt might be turning themselves on fantasizing about the cleaning lady or the mailman.

LAST WORD

The aim of this book was to show you just how much fun sex could be. I hope by reading this you have gone some way to overcoming any lingering shyness or embarrassment about the subject and picked out some ideas for putting some pizzazz into your sex life. Passion, romance, flirtation, fantasy, infatuation, excitement, lust, desire, moonlight and roses should be a part of everyone's relationship. This book was written to reassure you that it's your right and it's within your grasp, and to send you out to find it all in your relationship. The trick to having a good sex life is recognizing that we aren't born knowing how to arouse and satisfy ourselves, or how to do the same for a sexual partner. The only way you're going to learn is to set off on a journey of self-discovery, where you and your partner help yourselves to good loving and help each other to it, too. You don't have to be a health professional, knowing exactly how the body ticks, to learn how your own body and that of your partner jumps and twitches. All you need is the desire to find out, and the realization that it's OK to try.

Most of us are the best experts on our own love lives, if we've acquired the confidence to do the research. All it needs is for us to get down and dirty with the one we love, and to know that doing so is fine. This book was written to help you expand your own individual fantasy life, and help you bring this out to enhance your sexual relationship. Whether you go on from here to lighting a few candles occasionally and massaging each other with aromatherapy oils, or to spending every weekend in full dominatrix regalia, it really doesn't matter. What matters is that you get the love life that you deserve, which is the sex life you want. The only rule is "do no harm" to anyone else or yourself. And enjoy!

INDEX

Page numbers in *italic* indicate illustrations.

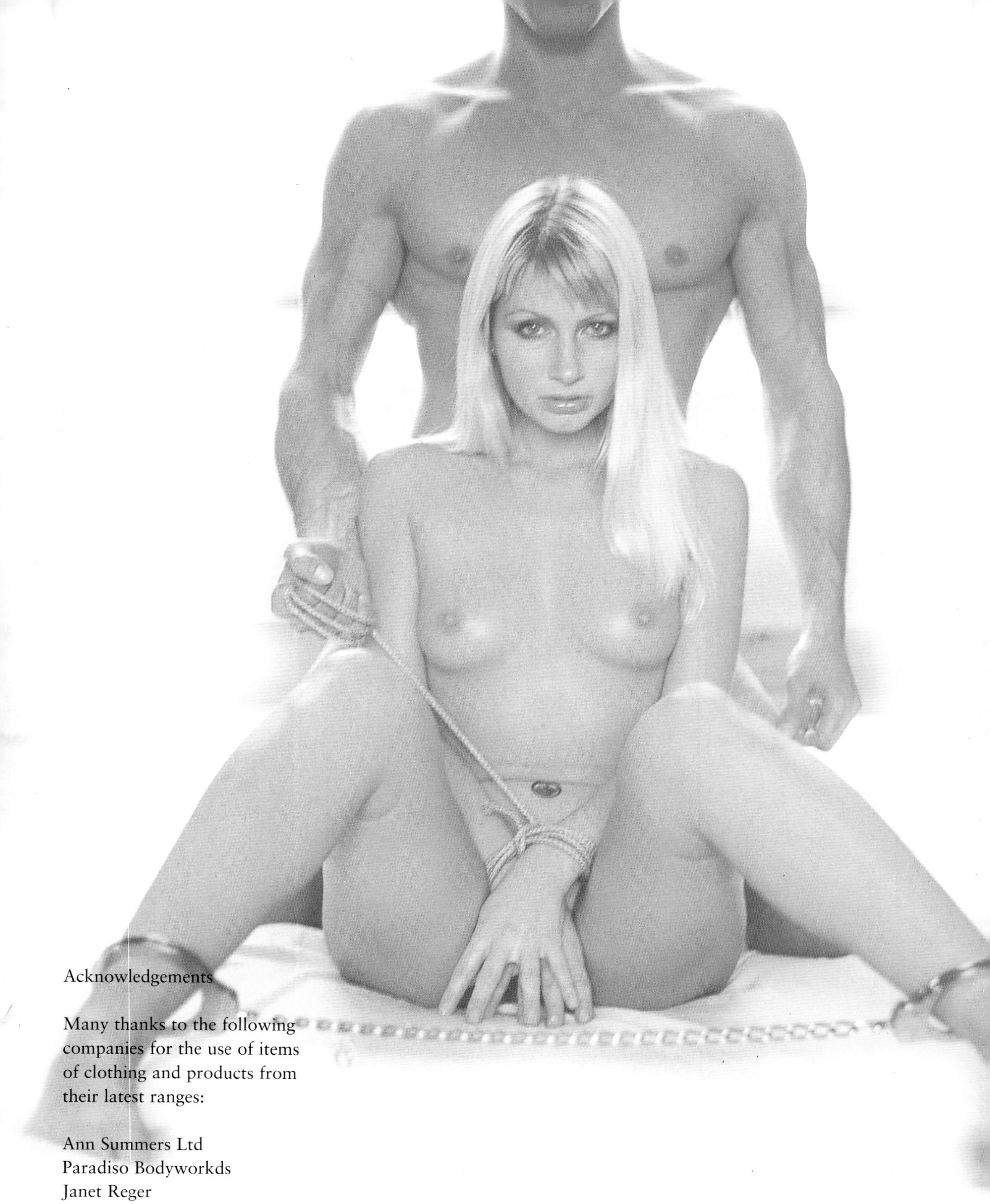

Acknowledgements

Many thanks to the following companies for the use of items of clothing and products from their latest ranges:

Ann Summers Ltd
Paradiso Bodyworkds
Janet Reger
Zeitgeist Ltd